GREAT BODY FOR BUSINESS TRAVELERS

Health & Fitness for Men Who Travel for Business

PROGRESS: move forward or onward in space and time
"as his age progressed he became more
appreciative, respectful and empathetic."

Chris R. Rea

ReaShape

ISBN: 978-0-9903094-4-4

The nutritional and health information in this book is based on the author's experiences. It is intended only as a guide and is not meant to replace the advice of a physician, dietitian, physical therapist, or other health professional. Always seek competent professional help if you have concerns about the appropriateness of this information for you.

Printed in the United States of America.

For my brother.

Contents

Chapter 1: About Business Travel: Is It Bad, Really Bad, for Your Health?

"How can business travel be bad for my health?" you ask. Because it does sound improbable: the very idea of travel, after all, conjures up excitement, fun, and carefree days in a relaxing spot far from home.

Sure, you might lose your luggage. But a health risk isn't what comes to mind when you imagine yourself on a trip to Aruba, Cancun, or Hawaii.

Frequent business travel (FBT), though—that's an entirely different story.

As *The Wall Street Journal* noted in a traveler-beware article titled "Business Travelers Pack Extra Pounds, Insomnia, Stress," if you travel two or more weeks a month for your job, you could be at risk for a surprising range of physical ailments. And after several years on the road, those ailments could lead to serious chronic health conditions, besides. More specifically, reported the Journal, research shows a clear relationship between life as a "road warrior" and life as someone who suffers from diminishing health. One such study, conducted by Columbia University's Mailman School of Public Health with a whopping 13,000 subjects, found that as the number of monthly travel days rose, so did the statistical likelihood of obesity. When travel ate up twenty-one days each month or more, the chance of becoming obese was an astonishing 92 percent. It was, in other words, all but inevitable.

But that's only the beginning. Researchers also discovered that, with an increase in pounds of fat, there was a corresponding increase in the chance that chronic medical conditions would develop over time.

Those chronic ailments included heart disease, Type 2 diabetes, high blood pressure, high cholesterol, and the risk of some forms of cancer. Sounds pretty serious, right?

Unfortunately, there are even more health hazards associated with frequent business travel, or FBT. And while the main message of this book is that building and maintaining health and fitness is the best way to counteract all these FBT hazards, it's still a good idea to know what the entire landscape of health risks for business travelers looks like. So let's briefly visit each of these additional risks—from the most common, to the quite frequent, to those that belong in the realm of worrisome possibilities.

Jet Lag

First of all, every business traveler who engages in the kind of frequent travel that forces him to cross one or more time zones on a regular basis realizes that "jet lag" is no urban myth. It causes real symptoms, and they range from the highly annoying to the truly debilitating.

Whenever you enter a time zone you're physically unaccustomed to, your internal clock (the part of you that regulates body temperature, blood pressure, hormones, and the glucose in your bloodstream, as well as the sensations of thirst, hunger, and the need for sleep) gets confused.

Because the appearance of either daylight or nighttime arrives at a different time than what you're used to, your body clock (also known as the brain's hypothalamus) may jumpstart physical functions that other parts of your body are not prepared for—and the symptoms of jet lag kick in.

So what are those symptoms?

They vary from person to person, of course. And they also vary depending upon how many time zones you crossed, and in which direction your travel occurred (whether west to east, or east to west). But they comprise the symptoms of nearly every single health challenge, apart from weight gain, that make FBT so strenuous and hard to manage.

There's the sheer fatigue, to begin with. Having disturbed circadian rhythms (daily cycles of waking and sleeping) is very tiring to the body. And that disturbance mixes uncomfortably with the insomnia that often results from arriving at a new destination in full daylight, when your body was expecting the dark of night --because of the time at your departure location.

Then there are the emotional symptoms that being out of sync causes. Depending on your general disposition and physiology, you may feel anxious, depressed, irritable, angry, or confused. You may also feel dizzy and could suffer from temporary memory loss. Obviously, this does not make life easy if you are due at an important meeting within an hour or two of your arrival.

Alas, these aren't the only symptoms you may suffer from. You could have a wicked headache, partly due to dehydration, which occurs courtesy of the always-very-dry air on jetliners. And you may feel nauseated, find yourself sweating profusely, and have difficulty with physical coordination. In addition to all that, you could be suffering from various forms of gastro-intestinal distress (an overly acidic stomach, constipation, or diarrhea).

But wait—just when you thought things could hardly get any worse—there are even more health negatives.

If you have a chronic health condition of some kind, you may find that your usual symptoms have intensified. You could notice heartbeat irregularities, for instance. Or could find that your compromised immune system can't protect you from a cold or the flu, and you arrive at your destination feeling sick.

Frequent business travel is certainly not for the less than physically robust.

The one ray of hope business travelers have is that all these jet lag symptoms are temporary. Full recovery usually takes a day for each time zone crossed (though symptoms are typically worse when more than two zones disappear beneath the wings of your plane). Your symptoms could also worsen when your trip entailed traveling from west to east, since time is lost and not gained, as it is when flying from east to west. (Noon on the east coast, for instance, in the eastern time zone, is just nine in the morning on the west coast, in the pacific time zone. So after a six-hour trip, you'll still arrive in Los Angeles three hours earlier than the time in New York, your departure city.)

But even the worst symptoms of jet lag should subside after a few days, leaving you only a bit more tired, perhaps, than you were when you started out, yet relatively symptom free.

Stress

Unfortunately, much of the above fallout from jet lag can descend upon business travelers, once again, in the form of stress. It isn't just physical stress, either; there is a psychological and emotional component. But because there is, it means that stress is something over which travelers can exert a certain measure of control.

For instance, if you notice that your anxiety level is beginning to rise because your taxi is stuck in traffic on the way to the airport—where your departing flight is scheduled to leave on the hour—you can take steps to calm yourself, thereby reducing your overall level of stress.

Of course, the causes of stress for frequent business travelers are rarely that simple. They tend to occur as a result of multiple rather than single triggering events. Most frequently, business travelers report that their stress comes from being concerned about family members back home, when forced to travel on short notice, and feeling pressured to accomplish sometimes unreasonable amounts of work without the office support that's available in the home office. This combination of factors can create a build-up of anxious feelings that can lead to physical and psycho-emotional tension and worse.

There's also the less-often-mentioned stress of isolation—being alone in strange surroundings, dealing with the challenges of speaking a language not one's own, and, at the end of the day, facing the loneliness of an impersonal hotel room. Inevitably, these emotional and psychological stressors translate into physical symptoms, in the form of headaches, emotional ups and downs, stiff necks, and tense shoulders.

And, in fact, a variety of studies, including one reported in the *International Journal of Stress Management,* found that frequent business travelers had psychological well-being scores that were quite a bit below the norm. Naturally, that impacts their job performance as well as their health. (Not surprisingly, frequent business travelers filed claims for psychological treatment at a rate three times that of those who did not travel for their job.)

Stress, for frequent business travelers, is real—not a partially imaginary feature of their work lives—and we'll look at ways to counteract it in upcoming chapters.

Poor Nutrition

If psychological stress can create physical stress, then poor nutrition—meals that are high-fat, high-carbohydrate (refined carbs, that is), high-calorie, and highly processed— affect more than your body. They affect your overall psychological well-being, too.

But when you're contemplating high-pressure business situations, your overall well-being naturally includes feeling and looking your best—something that can prove elusive for frequent business travelers.

Why is that?

Remember the research cited at the beginning of this chapter? The study which found that FBT led to a statistical probability for obesity of 92 percent? That finding correlates directly to the fact that business travelers are almost always either rushing around or waiting around in airports, or else sitting for hours on airplanes—two public environments that offer fast food in abundance. (For those who spend their travel time in cars, the same condition applies: every major interstate is littered with fast-food establishments.) All three of those travel environments offer few, if any, healthy, nourishing, and sustaining meal choices.

So it's easy to see how business travelers fall into the fast-food trap.

When they are rushing to catch a flight, the easiest and, indeed, the only nutritional option (apart from bringing their own breakfast, lunch, or dinner) is to grab some airport "faux food." Likewise, if their plane is delayed and they must wait in the airport lounge for hours, there's plenty of fast food but little else. Then once they're seated on their plane, the only food choices will be highly caloric, laden with salt, full of saturated fat (by some estimates, as much as 45 percent, and so processed that all nutritional value has long since vanished.

This abundance of airport, airline, and interstate fast food—with few if any other options—is the major business travel "ingredient" that has led, almost inevitably, to that frightening statistic for FBT obesity.

Though let's not forget one thing more: the role that alcohol plays in adding "empty" or non-nutritious calories to a business traveler's diet. For many, the stress of work while traveling internationally, and the pressure to socialize with business contacts in the evening, can add up to thousands of added calories (not to mention quite a few hangovers) from drinks on the plane, with dinner, and in the evening.

It only takes a few years of FBT before fast food and alcohol-fueled socializing add up to significant weight gain (enough to qualify as obesity—by definition, when body fat constitutes a third of a man's weight).

No Exercise

But fast food alone is rarely responsible for a weight gain so pronounced that it qualifies as obesity. Almost always, it's the combined effect of unhealthy food and little or no exercise, on business trip after business trip, year after year, that leaves a frequent business traveler feeling—and looking—his absolute worst.

It's true that business travel offers few naturally occurring opportunities for exercise. A business traveler could easily sit for twelve hours or more at a barely uninterrupted stretch. Starting with several hours in the airport lounge, sitting will continue with hours and hours on an international flight, followed by hours more in meetings immediately upon arrival, and end with an evening spent sitting around a restaurant table with business contacts.

Since meetings are often tightly scheduled to make the most of a business traveler's trip, there will be little time not devoted to work. And, on the return flight, it will be the same sedentary routine all over again.

So what does so much sitting and so little exercise do to a frequent business traveler's health? Pretty much the same thing it does to office workers who sit at a desk for six hours or more each workday. After a decade or two of sedentary work, they will have a 64 percent greater risk of heart disease, a 30 percent greater risk of prostate cancer, and can expect to subtract seven years from their life expectancy.

Of course, there's even more fallout from constant physical inactivity than the above three statistically measured outcomes.

Generally speaking, what sitting for prolonged periods does is to instigate a loss of physical stamina and strength, as well as a marked decline in optimal physical function. Muscles begin to atrophy after as little as two weeks of sitting. Cholesterol rises along with blood sugar, as the body becomes insulin resistant—all while the muscles, due to lack of use, fail to consume the body's stored fat. Even the lungs are affected: their maximum capacity for oxygen consumption declines, making exertion more difficult and, as a result, less appealing.

For frequent business travelers, though, there is one additional worry: "Traveler's Thrombosis." Sitting for prolonged periods of time under cramped conditions on an international flight can, for some people, cause such sluggish circulation in their legs that a blood clot may form, causing pain, redness, and swelling. The condition can become life threatening if part of the clot breaks off and migrates to the lungs, triggering a stroke. Fortunately, pulmonary embolism, as this is called, is relatively rare. It occurs in about one out of every one thousand travelers. But when you consider how many business travelers there are—in the neighborhood of five or six million in the U.S., in any given year since 2000—one in one thousand is a not insignificant number.

In the end, though, the worst health hazard that frequent business travelers face may be a simple lack of information—the hazard that comes from being uninformed. Many business travelers have only a vague idea of why cycling through jet lag, stress, poor nutrition, and lack of exercise for weeks at a time, month after month, year after year, is hazardous to their health and longevity. In fact, it's quite possible to feel poorly on a regular basis but not take it seriously—or not seriously enough. Ignorance, however, about the risks of FBT is most definitely not bliss.

So it's important to realize that whenever the human body doesn't get what it needs—whether rest, recreation (a stimulating variety of activities), good nutrition, or exercise— it reacts in the same way. There is a decline in overall health and functioning, followed by the onset of chronic and sometimes fatal conditions.

Given that bleak but logical outcome, the welcome news is that it's relatively simple to start nurturing your body with the things it needs to feel healthy and vibrantly alive, so it can perform in an optimal way. In fact, it could be considered an important job qualification. Physically fit, well-nourished business travelers can think clearly, react intelligently, and make good business decisions; they are an asset to themselves and their companies.

What Can Exercise Do for You?

The real question is: "What can't exercise do for you?"

There's almost no physical ailment or chronic condition that is caused by a sedentary lifestyle fraught with stress that does not respond to the transformative effect of daily exercise. Here are a few of the benefits you can expect.

Physical Benefits

Exercise reduces the likelihood of developing any number of chronic conditions because it improves overall health (compromised health is what allows chronic health conditions to develop in the first place). If a chronic condition already exists, exercise can help reduce its symptoms, if not eliminate the condition entirely.

Chronic conditions that respond well to exercise as preventive, if not curative, include:

• Heart disease (and the possibility of stroke)
• High blood pressure (and the possibility of a stroke or heart attack)
• High cholesterol (which increases the risk of heart disease)
• High blood sugar (and insulin resistance that can lead to type 2 diabetes)
• Osteoarthritis (stiffness and pain in joints)
• Osteoporosis (weak bones and low bone density)
• Cancer (certain forms, like prostate, colon, lung, and others)
• Obesity (when one third or more of the total bodily weight comes from fat)

Exercise can reduce the likelihood of weight gain, and help speed up weight loss, especially when combined with good nutrition.

Exercise can alleviate or prevent various forms of gastrointestinal distress, including bloating, an overly acidic stomach, constipation, and diarrhea.

Exercise can restore a healthy sleep patterns and reduce, if not eliminate, insomnia due to a travel-related disruption of the circadian rhythms.

Mental Benefits

Exercise can create the necessary "physiological foundation" for fast, clear thinking in situations demanding complex, difficult decisions—because it increases blood flow and oxygen, both of which directly nourish the brain, thus giving your mind what it needs to function optimally.

Exercise can actually help grow a larger brain, by encouraging the growth of new neurons; in fact, the more physically fit a person is, the larger the hippocampus tends to be, an area of the brain associated with spatial memory.

Exercise can make it easier to give up addictions like smoking, as the rewards of exercise serve to re-program the "reward pathways" in the brain, returning them to their original non-addicted setting.

Emotional Benefits

Exercise can mitigate feelings of anxiety, tension, and overall stress, because it decreases the presence of cortisol in the bloodstream. Cortisol is a hormone the body releases naturally in response to stress, but when stressful situations remain more or less constant, cortisol also remains high. Its chronic presence in the blood can cause a range of damaging physical effects, from muscle loss to weight gain. More immediately noticeable is the fact that cortisol can make it difficult to think clearly.

Strenuous exercise stimulates the release of endorphins, natural painkiller hormones (thought to be three times stronger than the drug morphine) that produce a feeling of physical happiness and well-being—a sense of elation that is like a natural high (the so-called "runner's high" comes from the release of endorphins).

Exercise also increases the level of serotonin present in the brain, a hormone that acts like an opiate to elevate mood and boost self-confidence. Serotonin is thought to be a natural antidepressant, one that can relieve depression, anxiety, and insomnia.

Along with the above results, exercise acts as an effective way to release accumulated tension and frustration, relaxing tense muscles and burning off negative emotions.

What Can Good Nutrition Do for You?

Exercise and good nutrition are the two legs you need to stand on, when enhancing or maintaining your optimal level of health and fitness. But, just as there are many systems for exercise, there are many perspectives about the best way to achieve nutritional balance.

That said, nutritional experts of all kinds seem to agree that the typical airport and airline fast-food diet (one featuring high-fat, high-carbohydrate, high-sugar, high-salt, high-calorie, highly chemicalized, and highly processed faux food) is not only a prescription for poor health, but, over time, for the development of chronic illnesses.

So what is good nutrition?

To begin with, and as you might expect, it is the opposite of fast food, in every respect. In other words, it is low-fat; low-simple-or-processed carbohydrates (complex carbs, on the other hand, are recommended); low-sugar; low-salt; low-calorie (but high in nutrients); non-chemicalized; not overly processed real food.

In short, it's the difference between an organically grown apple with roasted but unsalted organic almonds as a snack, and an order of fast-food-chain, highly salted, fat-laden French fries in a greasy paper sleeve (the kind of fries that, if left on a shelf for two months, would still look nearly the same—as if they were not food at all but an inert substance, a food "product").

Good nutrition also takes into account the fact that there are nutrients in close to the-way-nature-made-them foods that have not yet been discovered. In other words, good nutrition understands that "nature knows best." She designs vegetables, fruits, grains, beans, seeds, nuts, and sources of lean protein (in other words, animal products without antibiotics and growth hormones) in a way that is far more nutritionally complex than our current understanding can grasp. And in a way that is completely nourishing to human bodies.

Good nutrition allows food to be food—to do what it does best for our health and well-being. Here are some of its benefits.

Physical Benefits

Like exercise, good nutrition prevents the gradual development of common chronic conditions (diabetes, heart disease, hypertension, high cholesterol, arthritis, osteoporosis, obesity, stroke, cancers), at the same time that it nourishes all parts of the body at every level, from the smallest cell to the thirty- to forty-foot intestinal tract.

Good nutrition gives the body what it needs to grow new cells and repair itself, while maintaining all its functions at an optimal level. Quite simply, the body will become sicker and sicker and eventually die, without good nutrition.

Mental Benefits

The brain works best when the body works best. Good nutrition keeps the arteries flexible as well as free of fat deposits or plaque—so the blood which nourishes the brain (the one organ that requires more blood and oxygen than any other, in order to feed its 400 billion capillaries) flows freely.

When the brain is well-nourished, the cognitive functions on which we depend are not impaired; in fact, they're enhanced, and we can think clearly and quickly.

Emotional Benefits

Good nutrition tends to prevent the common business traveler complaint of mood swings. This is because the blood chemistry, instead of vacillating wildly due to the ingestion of toxic substances (from fast food), tends to remain more stable, since healthy food is not toxic.

Depression, while it can have many causes, is made worse by poor food choices, particularly choices that are high in sugar. But when nutrition is good or even excellent, depression tends to lift, as if the body's very cells then have the strength to feel optimistic again, because they are well-nourished.

Nutrition is vital to everyone. But for frequent business travelers, the physical, mental, and emotional demands of working while on the road are multiplied many times over. And so the need for each businessman to nourish his body with all the nutrients it requires for optimal functioning is that much greater, that much more important—for health and longevity.

How Travel/Fit Works

The Travel/Fit program is designed for three main types of frequent business traveler.

The first type, called the "Start-up Hero," is someone who needs to start practicing fitness and health with the basics. He needs to build his strength and stamina gradually, month after month, until he can safely graduate to the next level.

But make no mistake. The Start-up Hero really is a hero. It takes far more courage to begin exercising and eating healthier meals if you've neglected both for a long time, than it does if you've been conscientious about your health all along.

To create a clear picture of someone who is starting out at this level, we'll follow the progress of a typical business traveler, who we'll call Bob. He begins the program with twenty extra pounds, an aversion to exercise, and a love of fast food, beer, and anything sweet. Bob is pre-diabetic (type 2 diabetes) and has incipient heart disease, although he's not been diagnosed, yet. He is afraid to visit his doctor.

Bob will follow the Travel/Fit exercise and healthy food plan for his level, the Start-up Hero, and we'll watch him make progress, step by step, gradually but steadily.

If your current level of fitness is a bit like Bob's, his example will give you an idea of what's possible, the best way to approach working toward a new level of health and fitness, and what to expect along the way.

The next type of business traveler in the Travel/Fit program is the Entrepreneur. At this level, our typical businessman—who we'll call Dave—is either not overweight at all, or only has five pounds to lose. He's also someone who exercises regularly, if informally and a little sporadically, when he's not traveling. Dave knows that fast food makes him feel terrible after a few days of nothing but. So he tries to avoid it.

As with our previous fitness type, if your overall level is closer to Dave's, then watching him follow the Travel/Fit program for maintaining and enhancing his health and fitness will show you how to approach an effective on-the-road maintenance program of your own.

The third type of business traveler in the Travel/Fit system is the CEO. At this level, our typical businessman, who we'll call Ed, is a dedicated fitness and health buff. Traveling doesn't encourage him to put exercise on the back burner; far from it. Ed knows that the more challenging and stressful his trip is, the more he needs to exercise in order to restore his equilibrium and his ability to get work accomplished.

Ed may not be concerned with looking like the young Arnold Schwarzenegger, or winning weight-lifting contests, but his stamina and strength are unusual among his peers. His real secret is that he feels good living in his skin, almost all the time. For that, his exercise and healthy eating habits can be thanked, and he considers them non-negotiable.

If you're a bit like Ed, the Travel/Fit program will help you refine your exercise routine, suggest alternatives, and assist you in planning healthy eating on the road.

For Bob, Dave, and Ed—and you, whichever type you most resemble—motivation to exercise and eat healthy meals comes from noticing that you feel so much better when you do.

Nothing is more rewarding than getting to the point where you look forward to exercise, and really prefer the enjoyment of eating in a healthy way—other than, perhaps, walking through your front door after a long international trip.

Why I Wrote This Book

While I've traveled around the world for business, I am not a frequent business traveler. And yet, whenever I found myself on an international flight, I couldn't help but notice the multitude of business people populating so many of the surrounding seats.

When I saw businessmen who looked fatigued and harried, I wondered what steps they ought to be taking to achieve health and fitness. How would they find a way to fit exercise and good nutrition into their travel schedule?

And when I saw one of the relatively few men who did look fit, I wondered if he would eventually discover a way to maintain his health while traveling—whether he'd make the time.

After looking into the studies and statistics that had been compiled on the health of frequent business travelers, I realized that their predicament was a lot like mine when I had a motorcycle accident at age twenty-two.

Up until that accident, I'd been obsessed with working out every day, building muscle, maintaining optimal health, all in order to compete in weight-lifting contests and engage in the sports I loved to play. Being fit was a way of life that made me feel great.

But after I broke my sternum and several bones in my right hand, as well as my jaw, also losing several teeth—and suffered a collapsed lung, many lacerations, internal bleeding, and a damaged liver—it took me months to heal my internal injuries and broken bones. And during those months, I wasn't able to exercise at all. I soon lost muscle weight and gained "flab," while watching my usual feeling of vitality and strength drain away.

I was miserable; I no longer felt like myself. And I especially missed the daily endorphin high I got from vigorous exercise—the lift it gave me, the feeling of optimism that I could accomplish anything I might want to do.

It occurred to me that this was exactly how frequent business travelers feel: out of shape, tired and irritable, and lacking in the essential vitality that I'd always counted on for a daily sense of joie de vivre, that spark of joy in just being alive.

So it hit me: I had a lot of experience helping men achieve fitness and health. I'd coached friends, first, and later on, clients, for years. And I could use that experience to help business travelers achieve better fitness and improve their overall health. I decided to start with male business travelers since I know how men think and what they need. For instance, I understand that—while there are many exceptions—men in general tend to ignore health issues for a long time. And when they do decide to get fit, they tend to overdo it, trying to get in shape overnight. Not a wise idea.

Getting men to see that "slow and steady wins the race" is a major challenge, but one that I'm familiar with, since I have the same struggle with myself. In other words, the male tendency toward aggressiveness needs to be channeled constructively when it comes to creating fitness.

I also decided that I'd eventually partner with a female fitness expert who had lots of experience helping other women achieve fitness and health. Together, we'd develop a Travel/Fit system designed for women executives who are frequent business travelers.

Right now, though, I'd focus on working with men who travel frequently for business.

What You Can Expect

In the next three chapters, you'll learn how to improve your health and fitness, even if you've neglected both for years. And if you're already a fan of health and fitness and what it can do for you, you'll learn how to create routines for the road that help you maintain, if not enhance, your current levels.

The relatively small amount of extra effort involved will be returned to you a thousand fold in the form of overall well-being, physical health, and the kind of optimal mental performance that allows you to do your job with excellence, even when facing the unavoidable challenges of frequent business travel.

Chapter 2: The Health and Fitness Start-up Hero: Small Changes, Big Difference

It's easy to change an unhealthy habit. You just need to do an end-run around your amygdala.

". . . an end-run around my what?" you ask.

You know—that part of your midbrain that controls your "fight or flight" survival instinct. Also the part that produces fearful thoughts whenever you try to change your daily routine for the better.

Want to get up at 5:30 a.m. to fast-walk around your hotel's parking lot? "Sorry," says your amygdala (pronounced ah-MIG-duh-luh), "no can do. Not your usual morning routine. Probably dangerous! Stay in bed where you're safe."

What's Your Amygdala Got to Do With It?
Your amygdala floods your system with irrational thoughts like those above—fearful thoughts that try to pass themselves off as common sense. And the reason it does this is because it's your amygdala's job to keep you firmly cemented within the safety of your current comfort zone. Something it does exceedingly well.

So you can see what you're up against.

The task is not, as you might have thought, crawling out of bed while it's still dark, jumping into your sweats, and quietly making your way downstairs and through the hotel's revolving front door, whereupon you breathe the bracing fresh air as you fast-walk in the pre-dawn light.

No. It's much harder than that.

Your task is to fool your amygdala into thinking that the changes you want to make are not only completely safe, but no big deal. That they are, in fact, utterly normal behavior for you.

Think that sounds unlikely, if not impossible? Fortunately, it is not. Here's all you need to do:

Bypassing your mind's fearful thoughts is easy—if you start small. And you start small by taking tiny, tiny steps. Steps so tiny your amygdala doesn't notice what you're doing. And, as a result, its fear mechanism doesn't get activated; it continues to "sleep." (There is more neuroscience behind this tiny-step technique, and we'll look at that in just a few minutes.)

Back to your early-morning fast walk. In order to not set off an alarm in your amygdala, you need to spend three to four weeks doing what may seem like small-step tasks that lead nowhere. But, despite the way they seem, these tiny steps do lead to big changes in behavior—lasting changes, unlike overly ambitious efforts that later get abandoned because they're too difficult to sustain.

A Small-Step Scenario

Here, for example, is one possible small-step scenario (you can easily invent your own, once you see how it works).

Day One. Put your running shoes, socks, T-shirt, shorts, sweats, and baseball cap on a chair in your hotel room. Set your alarm for 5:30 a.m., or about an hour earlier than usual. When the alarm rings the next morning, get up, sit on the edge of your bed, and simply look at your running or walking clothes. (If you're easily bored, you can also pick each item up and put it back down. Nope, not kidding about that.) After ten minutes, set your alarm for the time that you really do need to get up, and go back to sleep.

Day Two. Do the same thing that you did on Day One. Notice whether you are beginning to feel a little impatient to put your sweats on and get outside. Tamp your impatience down, re-set your alarm, and get back to sleep.

Day Three. Same as Day One and Two. This time, though, visualize putting on your sweats, walking down the hall, getting on the elevator, walking across the lobby, exiting through the front door, and striding out into the parking lot or onto the hotel grounds. Then set your alarm as usual, and go back to sleep.

Day Four. Same as Day One, Two, and Three. Except, this time, try to imagine the experience of being outside in the pre-dawn light as a sensory experience. Breathe the fresh air. Feel the little thrill of being the only person awake at this time of day. Hear the few birds that have begun to chirp. Then set the alarm, and get back to sleep.

Day Five. Same as Day One, Two, Three, and Four. But this time, imagine yourself either walking quickly or jogging on the grounds of your hotel. Feel the oxygen as it enters your lungs, feel the muscles in your legs moving you along, feel your heart beat a little faster and your body warm up and even begin to sweat a little, as you move faster on the return stretch. Then set the alarm, and go back to sleep.

Day Six. By now you know the routine. This time, though, stand up and put on your running or walking clothes. Then sit on the edge of your bed and visualize yourself being outside in the early morning, running or walking on the hotel grounds. After ten minutes, set the alarm and go back to sleep.

Day Seven. Repeat everything you did on Day Six.

Day Eight. Again, repeat the previous day's routine.

Day Nine. Same as usual except, this time, walk out into the hallway, close the door to your room, pocket your keycard, and walk to the elevator. Once there, turn around and go back to your room. Set the alarm, and go to sleep.

Day Ten. Repeat the steps in Day Nine.

Day Eleven. If you can do so without alerting your amygdala, once you get to the elevator, go down to the lobby. If you start to have a fear response, turn around and go back to your room.

Day Twelve. Repeat Day Eleven.

Day Thirteen. If you can get to the lobby with no fear, find a comfortable chair and sit there for about fifteen minutes, preferably while looking outside at the pre-dawn light. Then return to your room, set the alarm, and go to sleep.

Day Fourteen. Same as Day Thirteen.

Day Fifteen. This time, when you get to the lobby (if you feel no fear), walk outside and stride across the parking lot or onto the grounds. Don't go far. After ten minutes, turn around and return to your room. Set the alarm, and go to sleep.

Day Sixteen. Repeat Day Fifteen.

Day Seventeen. Repeat Days Fifteen and Sixteen.

Day Eighteen. For the next seven days, very gradually expand the size of the territory you cover, as you either walk or jog in the early morning light. When you are spending thirty minutes or more outside, you may want to skip going back to sleep again, and just go into your usual morning shower and shave routine.

This very gradual acclimation process will take twenty-five or more day—nearly an entire month—to complete. But once you've gone through the process, you'll have habituated yourself to a healthy routine that would have been impossible to establish otherwise.

It would have been impossible because, if you'd suddenly leapt into a drastic change in your morning routine, your amygdala would've made you feel fearful and stressed. Not only that, but exercising too much—out of the blue—is a sure way to make that exercise unsustainable for very long. Big, sudden changes don't last.

Quick note: You could also go through your acclimation process in the evening before dinner; or when you first arrive at your destination after a long flight; or in the middle of the day between meetings. The best time is whenever you can fit it in, on a regular basis. Later on, you'll replace your acclimation process with your fitness routine, so you want to establish a flexible but regular schedule for first one and then the other.

The Science Behind Small Steps

Why do small steps work to create sustainable change?

In Dr. Robert Maurer's book, *One Small Step Can Change Your Life: The Kaizen Way,* this clinical psychologist and professor at the UCLA School of Medicine and the California Health & Longevity Institute explains it this way: "By taking small steps, you effectively rewire your nervous system [creating] new connections between neurons, so that the brain enthusiastically takes over the process of change and you progress rapidly toward your goal."

In other words, tiny steps do three important things: 1. They stimulate your brain in a non-threatening way; 2. They give your brain the time it needs to gradually create the neural pathways to support your new exercise routine; 3. And they do all that without triggering your amygdala's fear response.

Fear, as you've probably noticed, is counterproductive for change. When we're afraid, we can't think, can't be creative, can't do much of anything except "fight or flight"—which is exactly how fear is designed to operate within that very shrewd neural wiring that is our survival instinct.

That said, though, it's true that many of us contemplate making big changes in our lives because we are fearful for some reason. This is exactly what happened to our Health an Fitness Start-up Hero, who we'll call Bob.

Bob, the Health and Fitness Start-up Hero

After half a dozen years on the road, two or three weeks each month, Bob's annual physical (mandated by his company) frightened him into taking action. Not only was he twenty-five pounds heavier than when he first started this job, Bob now had higher blood pressure, higher cholesterol, and elevated blood sugar. He was on his way to hosting several serious chronic conditions at once. My trifecta, he thought, feeling glum.

"But it's not too late to reverse these illnesses," his doctor told him. "Ditch the fast food. Lose weight. Get yourself a personal trainer. And learn how to de-stress in a healthy way. Cut way back on the alcohol. It's not a real way to relax, and it's doing you no good."

Bob immediately agreed to do better with his diet and start exercising, but he was secretly shocked. His whole life, he'd been nothing but healthy. He played high school and college basketball—and was no bench-warmer, either. Even just three years ago, he was known for his killer spike shot among the couples who gathered to play volleyball each summer at the beach.

How could he now be on the verge of having such middle-aged illnesses as high blood pressure, high cholesterol, and even diabetes? What had he done to bring this on himself?

Was it all that unhealthy food? Bob visualized the mountains of burgers and fries that he must have consumed. The armloads of doughnuts. The hundreds, maybe thousands, of cups of coffee with half 'n half and sugar. The sea of expense-account steak dinners. The boatload of creamily caloric desserts. The three or four drinks each evening (could they really add up to a thousand or so, each year?).

But everyone he knew ate that way on the road. There were guys out there who were much more overweight than he was—guys who probably didn't have a clue that "healthy eating" even existed.

"Come back in about four months, Bob," his physician said. "If you can, eat better. Stick with vegetables and fruits, whole grains, beans, seeds, nuts, and lean protein. And if you can get regular exercise, at least thirty minutes a day, I think we can avoid putting you on drugs for the hypertension and high cholesterol. Those meds have serious side effects, and you don't want to go that route if you can avoid it."

"Okay," Bob said, but he was thinking, In four months, I'll be in such good shape you won't believe your eyes. I'm not some chubby guy who needs four drinks to get to sleep. I can play b-ball, still. You'll see.

Fear sometimes masquerades as anger. And Bob chose to bury his fear by being covertly angry at his physician, adopting an "I'll show you" attitude. That anger propelled him into exercise like a racehorse pawing the ground at the starting gate. He took a week of vacation time to launch what he thought of as his "Get-Healthy-Quick Program."

On the first day—after his wife left for work, and his son and daughter were off at their summer camp jobs—Bob found a basketball in his garage and drove to the local high school. He'd take a few shots, jog around the school's track as many times as he could manage, then go home for sit-ups and pushups (no need to call attention to himself doing that in public). In the afternoon, he'd mow the lawn.

Bob felt completely optimistic. It was a beautiful summer day, not too hot, with a nice light breeze in the air. At the high school, there was one empty court—the others were being used by young kids—and Bob started taking shots. It felt good, watching the ball whoosh through the net and land with a smart bounce. But it didn't feel good to realize how fat he'd gotten. Not only that, but his blood was pounding in his temples after five or six shots. Maybe he'd just walk around the track.

This Bob did, and he completed ten circuits, mostly at a walk, before driving home. He figured that he'd done about three miles. In his living room, doing sit-ups and pushups, Bob made himself do two sets of five each, before collapsing on the rug, breathing hard. This was not going to be as easy as he'd thought.

During Bob's week off, he forced himself to make it around the high school track each day, logging three or four miles before driving home. He also forced himself to eat healthy meals—an egg on whole wheat toast, or else oatmeal with fruit, most mornings; and, say, bean salad or marinated tofu with asparagus and tomatoes for lunch; and usually a big green salad with a small piece of salmon for dinner. For dessert, he had watermelon and cantaloupe with raspberries and blueberries. Also, no alcohol at all—just unsweetened ice tea as an evening drink.

It wasn't too bad. He could do this. Besides, he felt thinner, even if the scale said that he weighed nearly the same.

The following week, Bob was back at work and about to fly to San Francisco to meet with new clients. He found it too hard to make breakfast before commuting to work, so he skipped that meal and gulped four cups of coffee, black, to get through the morning. By lunchtime, he was starved, but only had fifteen minutes between client calls to scarf something down. He grabbed a burger and fries in the food court of his office building, since it was the quickest, most familiar option.

On the plane the next day, Bob ate the airline food, and in the evening went out to dinner with his new clients. He couldn't not drink; they did. He couldn't not have steak; the fish would make him look "weak." And so it went. In under a week, Bob had abandoned his program, and was back to eating poorly and exercising not at all.

It didn't have to be that way. All Bob needed was a doable plan for building and maintaining his health and fitness level, one that would work despite the travel demands of his job. Instead, Bob put his energy into showing his doctor that he wasn't some unhealthy, overweight guy on his way to a stroke. But that goal ceased to be very motivating once Bob's usual routine resumed.

Fortunately, he got a second chance. A month after Bob went back to fast food and returned to his sedentary lifestyle, he got on the bathroom scale and realized that he'd gained nearly seven additional pounds. His self-esteem rebelled, demanding that he do something—even if it meant hiring a personal trainer, as his doctor had suggested.

Not Entirely Bob's Fault

We'll get back to Bob's health and fitness story in just a bit, but there's something that should be pointed out first. While it's true that Bob made consistently unhealthy choices since beginning his travel-intensive job, six years before, his declining health wasn't entirely his fault. There were several larger factors at work. So let's explore a few of those factors, the ones most dangerous to the health of business travelers like Bob.

Trans Fat

Hydrogenated vegetable oil was invented in the early 1900s, but it wasn't until the 1950s that this man-made cooking oil—later known as "trans fat"—really took off. The artificially solidified oil, that gave food products a much longer shelf life than ever before, was added to fast food, snack food, and baked goods for the first time in that era (everything from fried chicken and French fries, to cookies, crackers, and chips, to doughnuts and apple pie).

But it took another four decades before a link between trans fat and obesity, heart disease, and diabetes was finally suspected and confirmed. As these highly detrimental consequences began to percolate into public awareness, the purveyors of fast food, and other foods containing large amounts of the deadly fat, began to disavow it. Public pressure had forced them to respond.

In 2007, for example, many major hotel chains in the United States informed their guests that they had eliminated all trans fats from the food they served. For frequent business travelers, that still leaves airports with their fast food emporiums, as well as the many restaurants that never stopped using trans fat. But it was a start.

So how does this man-made fat create chronic conditions like heart disease, diabetes, and obesity?

Partially hydrogenated vegetable oil, or trans fat, has the unique ability to raise the level of "bad," or LDL, cholesterol, while at the same time lowering the level of "good," or HDL, cholesterol. And an increase in "bad" cholesterol leads to plaque buildup, or fatty deposits on the walls of your arteries (also known as atherosclerosis), which in turn makes it difficult for blood to flow freely. When the arteries that supply your heart suffer from atherosclerosis, chest pain and related symptoms of coronary artery disease can occur. And should a plaque deposit rupture, it could result in a traveling blood clot. If that clot ends up blocking the flow of blood to your heart, a heart attack could be the result; if it blocks the flow of blood to your brain, it could cause a stroke.

Trans fat also increases the presence of triglycerides (which may harden arteries and increase the risk of stroke, diabetes, heart disease, and heart attack). And trans fat increases the presence of Lp(a) lipo-protein (which increases plaque buildup in the arteries). Trans fat may increase inflammation, as well (by damaging the cells lining the blood vessels, thus causing inflammation, which in turn stimulates fatty deposits).

The health risks posed by trans fat were and are sufficiently serious that, in 2006, the FDA finally made mandatory the labeling of foods containing this man-made substance. Somewhat alarmingly, though, the federal agency subsequently estimated that, by warning the public with food labeling, there would be a savings of between $900 million and $1.8 billion, annually, in medical costs, lost productivity, pain, and suffering. In other words, trans fat is thought to cause all of the above "damage" on an annual basis.

So what does all this mean for Bob?

His weight gain—like that of many other business travelers—is at least partially the result of consuming large amounts of trans fat over half a dozen years. And his incipient high cholesterol and heart disease are surely related to trans fat, too, as is his elevated blood sugar.

But that's only the beginning. There are other unhealthy ingredients lurking in the food that most business travelers routinely consume.

High-Fructose Corn Syrup

In the 1970s, enzymes were used to treat corn syrup, creating an extremely sweet syrup that was also extremely cheap. This new sweetener was less expensive than sugar, the substance it largely replaced in many varieties of processed food, and even meat, since it also acted as a preservative. As a result, high-fructose corn syrup (HFCS), the sweetener cheaper than sugar, made financially feasible the "super-size" trend in fast food.

The problem is, high-fructose corn syrup contains 10 percent more sugar, in the form of fructose, and hence 10 percent more calories than sugar. Its caloric damage is worse. And, because the body can only metabolize fructose through the liver, when there is excess (as there is with supersized servings of soda, say) all the fructose the liver can't use will be turned into fats—into triglycerides, which are harmful to the arteries and the heart. One thing more: HFCS has also been linked to a form of liver scarring known as non-alcoholic fatty liver disease (NAFLD). Supersize doesn't look so "super" after all.

More proof of that fact was provided by a Princeton University study reported in the journal, *Pharmacology, Biochemistry and Behavior*. This research found that rats fed HFCS for six months gained 48 percent more weight than rats that were not fed the sweetener.

It would seem that HFCS is yet another culprit among several that caused Bob to gain thirty-two pounds, become pre-diabetic, and develop both higher cholesterol and blood pressure. After six years of consuming the artificial sweetener in all kinds of processed food—fast food, airline food, restaurant food, even in food that wasn't sweet in the least, like salad dressing, this was the combined toll that high-fructose corn syrup consumption took on his health.

More Ingredients to Avoid

Unfortunately, trans fat and HFCS are not the only health-destroying ingredients found in the fare commonly available to business travelers. Most fast food and other restaurants use a buffet of additives, all of them harmful to human health.

Some of the most troubling additives fall under the category of neurotoxins, which means that they affect the neurological pathways of the brain.

MSG, the liberally used flavor enhancer, is known to turn off the brain's sensation of being full, by interfering with neurological pathways. (You can see how it would contribute to weight gain.) MSG can also cause depression, disorientation, eye damage, fatigue, and headaches.

Another common neurotoxin is aspartame (Nutra-Sweet, Equal), the so-called "sugar-free" sweetener found in diet sodas and other diet products. Aspartame is known to not only erode intelligence but to affect short-term memory. Its other side effects include: lymphoma, brain tumors, diabetes, multiple sclerosis, Parkinson's, Alzheimer's, fibromyalgia, chronic fatigue, depression, anxiety attacks, dizziness, headaches, nausea, mental confusion, and seizures.

Still more neurotoxic additives are represented by the preservatives, BHA and BHT. While they prevent foods from changing color and flavor or becoming rancid, they also form cancer-causing compounds in the human body, and are known to alter behavior, as well.

Then there are miscellaneous additives, all of them highly toxic in their own way. These include six kinds of food dye (found in candy, baked goods, cheese); sodium nitrate and sodium nitrite (found in processed meats); sulfur dioxide (found in beer, soda, fruit juice); and potassium bromate (found in bread and rolls).

The kicker is, the food industry has developed additives that not only make food taste better, they make eating such foods addictive (similar to the way that tobacco companies added chemicals to cigarettes to make smokers even more addicted to smoking than they already were).

A business traveler's only defense lies in taking individual responsibility for what he consumes on the road. In particular, that means making the effort to read labels and avoid food with trans fat, HFCS, and additives of any kind.

So What Can Business Travelers Eat?
Good question. No less an authority than the Department of Nutrition at the Harvard School of Public Health has an answer, one based on the latest scientific findings. That last nuance is important.

Harvard takes the USDA (United States Department of Agriculture) to task for publishing faulty dietary guidelines in 2011. After the federal agency replaced its old "food pyramid" illustrating what a healthy diet should look like with a new "plate" diagram, Harvard noted that the new USDA guidelines overlooked crucial elements because of political pressure from food industry groups.

As a result, Harvard's own food pyramid and food plate exist to correct misinformation provided by the USDA, and are "based exclusively on the best available science and [are] not subjected to political and commercial pressures from food industry lobbyists."

What's the difference between these two sets of guidelines?

The USDA, for one thing, doesn't distinguish between refined grains and whole grains. This is critical because white-flour foods quickly turn to sugar in the body; whole grains, however, are digested slowly and provide long-lasting energy that is less likely to become stored as fat. For another thing, the USDA recommends drinking milk with every meal, while Harvard recommends water (or tea or coffee). The reason is, in the first instance, the dairy lobby is quite influential with the USDA and that is a deciding factor. And, in the second instance, the reason is that Harvard finds no value in the claims made for dairy products but does recognize that "high intakes" of dairy increase the risk of cancer.

There are other differences, as well. Harvard, for instance, recommends what it calls healthy protein, which includes fish, poultry, beans, tofu, seeds, and nuts. But it suggests limiting the consumption of red meat and absolutely avoiding all processed meat (bacon, hot dogs, sausages, and the like). The USDA, not surprisingly, makes no distinction between healthy and unhealthy sources of protein.

Harvard recommends consuming lots of different vegetables and fruits, but does not recommend white potatoes or French fries. The USDA, though, makes no distinction between healthy vegetables and starchy carbohydrates like white potatoes and French fries. Harvard recommends healthy oils, or vegetable oils like olive or canola, while limiting butter and avoiding trans fats completely. The USDA, though, says nothing about healthy vs. unhealthy fats.

Finally, there's this difference: at the base of Harvard's food pyramid, staying active, or getting daily exercise, is recommended along with controlling weight through moderate food portions. But the USDA is silent on the role of exercise in health maintenance, and silent on the role of moderate food portions in maintaining a healthy weight.

What's the takeaway for someone like Bob?

The Harvard nutritional guidelines, as set forth in their "Healthy Eating Plate" and "Healthy Eating Pyramid," recommend a diet in which the largest portion of every meal (with the exception of breakfast) is comprised of vegetables, followed by whole grains, healthy oils, healthy protein, and accompanied by fruits and water.

Healthy protein, according to the Harvard guidelines, includes fish, poultry, eggs, beans, tofu, nuts and seeds. Healthy oils include vegetable oils like olive, canola, soy, and sunflower. Dairy products, however, should be limited to one or two small servings per day. Outright unhealthy foods such as red meat, processed meat, butter, refined grains and white rice, white bread, semolina pasta, white potatoes, sugary drinks, sweet, and salt are to be eaten sparingly, if at all. Alcohol, in moderation, is optional, but not recommended for everyone. A daily multivitamin and extra Vitamin D, on the other hand, is recommended for most people. You can learn more about the Harvard recommendations at hsph.harvard.edu/nutritionsource.

Making Healthy Eating Work on the Road

It's helpful to have clear guidelines about which foods to eat and which to avoid, in order to achieve and maintain optimal health. But there remains one big stumbling block for Bob and every frequent business traveler. How can anyone possibly find healthy food (as defined by the Harvard guidelines) at airports, on airplanes, or in hotel restaurants?

The short answer: They can't.

But the real answer to this question is that Bob and his fellow business travelers simply have to make their health a priority, rather than something that's near the bottom of their "to do" list or not on their radar at all. Once making their health a top priority, they can plan before each trip and find ways of obtaining healthy food in places that would seem to offer none.

And how might that work?

What Bob will need to do is find ways of taking food with him, buying it on the road, and locating restaurants in his destination city that offer the meals he needs (by searching on line before his trip).

Admittedly, careful planning is no piece of cake, given that a road warrior's work life is typically hectic and strenuous. But what's the alternative?

Living with chronic illnesses is far worse than planning to take along healthy snacks, buy some fruit and vegetables at a grocery store, and locate vegetarian restaurants in the city where you're staying for a week or more. Vegetarian restaurants tend to offer lots of delicious vegetable choices. I'm not a vegetarian by any means, but I enjoy eating at these restaurants.

In the next chapter, Chapter Three, we'll talk about ways that every business traveler can plan his meals before traveling, and how to locate resources for creating healthy meals.

For someone like Bob, though, who's just beginning to work on creating and maintaining his health and fitness while traveling, it's important to start with small steps. He could substitute broiled fish or chicken several times a week, instead of having steak nearly every night. And he could pack instant oatmeal to make in his hotel room (using boiling water from the coffeemaker provided in most rooms), rather than scarfing down two or three doughnuts for breakfast.

At the same time, Bob might begin training himself to eat six smaller meals each day: breakfast, mid-morning snack, lunch, mid-afternoon snack, dinner, evening snack. This is preferable to eating three big meals, or even two meals on the run, with one big meal at the end of the day (when it will be sure to keep him awake).

This six-small-meals strategy will also keep Bob's metabolism going strong and never dipping too low, so it will burn more stored fat. And it'll also do away with the mistake of waiting too long before eating. The reason waiting too long between meals is never a good idea is because when we're really hungry, our first inclination is to grab anything that looks good, whether it's healthy or not. So it's much easier to make healthier choices if we're not starving. Packing trail mix, or perhaps unsalted roasted organic almonds with unsulfurized organic raisins, figs, dried apricots, or dried cherries can be a lifesaver, in this regard. And even though nuts and dried fruit are fairly caloric, their nutritional value and fiber content are far greater than a candy bar or a cinnamon roll (which would be loaded with additives, besides).

As mentioned earlier, in Chapter Three we'll look at specific strategies for finding healthy food on the road, strategies that anyone— whether a Fitness Start-up Hero, an Entrepreneur, or a CEO—can use to stay healthy while traveling.

Bob Commits to Getting Fit

Of course, food isn't everything. It's only half of a whole health and fitness program, one that includes both healthy eating and healthy exercise.

And even though, as we saw earlier, Bob wasn't successful in establishing an exercise program that worked for him while on the road, he was so annoyed with himself for gaining weight and developing three incipient chronic illnesses—high blood pressure, high cholesterol, and elevated blood sugar—that he wanted to do whatever it took to get his physical health back. As a result, Bob bit the bullet and hired a personal health and fitness trainer. He was getting serious, at last.

The first thing Bob's new trainer did was ask about his most recent medical checkup. And because Bob had seen his doctor only a month ago, there was no need to schedule another physical. Even so, Bob's trainer, who we'll call Tom, listened carefully as Bob enumerated all the physical problems he was experiencing, along with his physician's diagnosis.

They would start off, Tom explained, with gradual diet substitutions (like those mentioned above) in combination with small steps toward a complete but doable exercise routine that Bob could do almost anywhere.

We'll take a look at the slow-and-steady fitness program Tom designed for Bob in just a minute, but let's first examine something even more fundamental to fitness than regular exercise. As we saw in Chapter One, sitting for hours and hours can be deadly for anyone, but especially for business travelers who are essentially imprisoned in an airline seat or car seat while traveling.

The reason sitting is so detrimental to your health is because the body reacts in specific, health-negative ways when you sit for extended periods. In essence, it begins to shut down at the metabolic level, which means that there is a cascading series of physiological events that, taken together, do a great deal of harm.

First, circulation slows down, and far fewer calories are used, while the enzymes that break down triglycerides (fat) switch off. After an entire day of sitting, fat-burning activity will be reduced by half.

Second, without movement, your body uses much less blood sugar and your chances of developing type 2 diabetes begin to rise. At the same time, your risk of heart disease shoots up because the fat-burning enzymes that control blood fats are, as mentioned above, "asleep."

Finally, as your circulation slows down, far fewer mood-elevating hormones circulate to your brain, and the result is what might be called "sitter's depression."

So, you may be thinking, I'll just exercise more and avoid all the consequences of sitting for hours. Alas, even if you work out for thirty minutes every single day without fail, it won't offset the damage that sitting does.

What you need to do, instead, is get up every twenty minutes or so, and stretch and move around for a short time. The idea is to give the large muscles in your legs the chance to "reset" your body's various functions by virtue of the leg muscle contractions that accompany walking and standing. If you do that, research shows that you can put a big dent in the long-term decline in your overall health that sitting for hours and hours, year after year, decade after decade, inevitably causes.

The Fitness Start-up Program

When Tom, Bob's new fitness and health trainer, designed a program that Bob could do on the road, he included three main types of exercise. Cardio (heart muscle) exercise. Strength (bones, musculoskeletal) exercise. And stretching (muscle flexibility) exercise. Together, cardio, strength, and stretching create a balanced workout, one that will help Bob achieve whole-body fitness, over time. Here's a little more information about how these three types of exercise work to create optimal health and fitness.

Cardiovascular Exercise

This type of exercise is strenuous enough to get the heart muscle pumping faster, in order to stimulate the entire circulatory system. Amped-up circulation, some experts say, is capable of opening up clogged arteries and veins. And the sweat that results from this level of exertion can rid the body of accumulated toxins.

But cardio can do a lot of other things, too. It can relieve stress, boost energy, prevent such diseases as high blood pressure, heart disease, type 2 diabetes, arthritis, and some cancers. And it can also assist in losing weight, relieving depression, and getting more restful sleep.

Strength Training Exercise

Lifting as well as pushing against weights—strength training—can strengthen and even thicken bones, skeletal muscle, and tendons and ligaments. It strengthens the heart, as well, allowing it to pump more efficiently and lower blood pressure.

There's more: lifting weights increases lean muscle mass, which raises your metabolic rate so you burn more calories, even when sitting. It can also reduce the symptoms of arthritis, back pain, depression, and diabetes. Finally, lifting weights can boost your self-confidence along with your stamina.

Stretching Exercise

As anyone who travels frequently knows, sitting and doing relatively little for five or six hours is exhausting. One way to counteract sitting fatigue is to get up and stretch every muscle you can find. Stretching relieves muscle tension and even emotional stress because it makes you feel more energetic. This is partly because stretching restores more healthful circulation, and partly because it increases the range of motion in the body's many joints.

Stretching can be done at any time—all day, every day (and night)—but it is especially important to stretch gently and fully before cardio exercise and before strength-training, as well as immediately following both. Maintaining your body's flexibility will reduce the chance of an exercise injury, and it will keep you limber, even while sitting for hours at a time.

Exercise Tools to Go

Before we take a look at the four-month fitness program that Tom designed for Bob, here are a few tools that the personal trainer suggested, in order to make Bob's slow-and-steady progress toward fitness easier and more enjoyable.

The first tool Tom recommended for Bob was an inexpensive, battery-powered pedometer. Wearing it clipped to the top of his sweatpants before outdoor cardio, or even clipped to his belt when he had time to walk in an airport, would allow Bob to know how far he'd walked, so he could measure his progress accurately. It would also give Bob a way to compete against himself (two miles yesterday; two and a half today; three tomorrow).

Since it's so easy to forget where and when we exercise while on the road, or even if we exercised yet this week, Tom suggested that Bob carry a small hardbound notebook in which to write down everything he did each day toward his health and fitness. All his exercises and everything he ate would appear in his fitness log, so he could see how he was doing and where he needed to go next.

Finally, since not every hotel has a gym on the premises, Tom suggested that Bob get a lightweight exercise tube. This is a length of rubber tubing, somewhat like a jump rope, that has a handle on each end. It comes in various levels or degrees of resistance to being pulled or stretched, and thus mimics the muscle-stressing effect of lifting weights, so it's used for strength-training exercises. (Weights are too heavy for a carry-on bag, but exercise tubing weighs very little.)

Bob's Four-Month Fitness Exercise Routine

Bob needed a fitness routine he could quickly do in a hotel room or office, without changing into gym clothes. He worked with his trainer to come up with exercises that were easy to do and didn't need any equipment. They worked out a four-month routine with weekly variations. The routine was designed to help Bob gradually move to a higher fitness level without taking a lot of time for each session. By following the routine almost every day, Bob found that he had a lot more stamina. He could carry his suitcase and briefcase through an airport terminal without noticing their weight; he got through his busy workdays and still had energy to spare for more work in the evening or to enjoy some time off.

Light Daily Workout

When you're traveling, you can't always work out much. Your hotel might not have a gym, or your schedule might not have time for long workout. The daily workout schedule below is designed to help you get into better shape over a four-month period. The exercises can all easily be done in your hotel room or in an office or conference room. No gym is needed--you can do these exercises without even taking off your tie. Aim for a regular daily routine, taking one day off a week. If you can't manage that, just aim to do the routine as many days as you can. Any amount of exercise is better than none. Once you get into this routine, you'll probably find that you feel a lot better and have more energy to get through the day. That's a great incentive to work out every day whenever possible.

If you're new to exercise, remember that good form is important for avoiding injury. To see how to do the exercises, check my ReaShape channel on YouTube. You can also search YouTube for videos posted by many other trainers or check bodybuilding.com for videos.

Month One
Week One

Pre-workout stretching	10 standing toe touches
Cardio exercise	20 jumping jacks
Stretching	10 standing toe touches
Strength training	20 standing push-ups
Post-workout stretching	10 standing toe touches

Week Two

Pre-workout stretching	10 neck twists
Cardio exercise	10 vertical jumps
Stretching	20 standing arm spins
Strength training	20 body squats
Post-workout stretching	20 standing arm spins

Week Three

Pre-workout stretching	10 seated toe touches
Cardio exercise	15 seconds jogging in place
Stretching	10 seated toe touches
Strength training	20 door jamb pulls
Post-workout stretching	10 circular hip turns

Week Four

Pre-workout stretching	10 standing Superman stretches
Cardio exercise	10-minute walk
Stretching	10 standing Superman stretches

Strength training	20 standing push-ups
Post-workout stretching	10 standing Superman stretches

Month Two

Week One

Pre-workout stretching	10 wide-stance bent-over hamstring stretches
Cardio exercise	20 jumping jacks
Stretching	10 wide-stance bent-over hamstring stretches
Strength training	20 body squats
Post-workout stretching	10 wide-stance bent-over hamstring stretches

Week Two

Pre-workout stretching	10 seated toe touches
Cardio exercise	5-minute walk
Stretching	10 seated toe touches
Strength training	20 door jamb pulls
Post-workout stretching	10 seated toe touches

Week Three

Pre-workout stretching	10 circular hip stretches
Cardio exercise	20 jumping jacks
Stretching	10 circular hip stretches
Strength training	20 standing push-ups
Post-workout stretching	10 circular hip stretches

Week Four

Pre-workout stretching	10 standing toe touches
Cardio exercise	15 seconds jogging in place
Stretching	10 standing toe touches

Strength training	20 body squats
Post-workout stretching	10 standing toe touches

Month Three

Week One

Pre-workout stretching	10 wide-stance circular hip stretches
Cardio exercise	10-minute walk
Stretching	10 wide-stance circular hip stretches
Strength training	20 door jamb pulls
Post-workout stretching	10 wide-stance circular hip stretches

Week Two

Pre-workout stretching	15 standing toe touches
Cardio exercise	30 jumping jacks
Stretching	15 standing toe touches
Strength training	25 body squats
Post-workout stretching	15 standing toe touches

Week Three

Pre-workout Stretching	15 standing Superman stretches
Cardio exercise	25 seconds jogging in place
Stretching	15 standing Superman stretches
Strength training	25 standing push-ups
Post-workout stretching	15 standing Superman stretches

Week Four

Pre-workout stretching	15 seated toe touches
Cardio exercise	10-minute walk

Stretching	15 seated toe touches
Strength training	25 door jamb pulls
Post-workout stretching	15 seated toe touches

Month Four
Week One

Pre-workout stretching	15 standing toe touches
Cardio exercise	25 vertical jumps
Stretching	15 standing toe touches
Strength training	25 body squats
Post-workout stretching	15 standing toe touches

Week Two

Pre-workout stretching	15 wide-stance hamstring stretches
Cardio exercise	25 seconds jogging in place
Stretching	15 wide-stance hamstring stretches
Strength training	25 standing inclined push-ups
Post-workout stretching	15 wide-stance hamstring stretches

Week Three

Pre-workout stretching	15 wide-stance circular hip stretches
Cardio exercise	30 jumping jacks
Stretching	15 wide-stance circular hip stretches
Strength training	25 door jamb pulls
Post-workout stretching	15 wide-stance circular hip stretches

Week Four

Pre-workout stretching	15 standing arm spins
Cardio exercise	30 seconds jogging in place
Stretching	15 standing arm spins
Strength training	25 body squats
Post-workout stretching	15 standing arm spins

How Did Bob Do?

After four months of regular exercise and healthier meals, during which Bob's progress was closely watched, and sometimes course-corrected, by his trainer, Tom, he was on his way back to health and fitness.

When Bob returned to his doctor for another physical, he learned that not only had he dropped ten pounds, but his blood pressure, cholesterol, and blood sugar had all dropped, as well. He still had between twenty and twenty-five more pounds to lose, but Bob intended to keep building his strength and overall fitness.

In fact, he told his doctor that his new goal was to get to a level of fitness that would put him among the healthiest men in his age group, statistically speaking. Bob knew that goal was within reach, he told his physician. All he needed was another four or five months. "Piece of cake—uh, tofu," he said, grinning.

Chapter 3: The Health and Fitness Entrepreneur: Taking It on the Road

Frequent business travelers are a unique tribe of businesspeople, in that they must develop an equally unique set of on-the-job survival skills. Not only must they teach themselves to be effective under pressures that their office-bound colleagues will never face, they must do so while learning how to cope with a quartet of travel-related conditions—conditions that can have a big impact on their health, well-being, and job performance.

The Frequent Business Travel Quartet

In Chapter One, we saw how this quartet—jet lag, stress, poor nutrition, and little or no exercise—can take a huge physical and mental toll. They do so, in part, because these travel-toll inevitabilities work together in a synergistic way, over time, to degrade a traveler's health and fitness. In other words, the combined effect of all four is far worse than any one of them alone.

But there's something else, too. This quartet of adverse conditions not only works synergistically over the long haul, it works synergistically in the immediate present. Jet lag increases stress, which increases the tendency to overeat highly caloric fare with little nutritional value, which in turn leads to no exercise. Who feels like doing cardio or strength training after consuming two whoppers, a large fries, and a supersize shake?

But there is a silver lining.

Synergistic Healthy Opposites

The very fact that there's a synergistic relationship among the worst side effects of business travel also means that there's a synergistic relationship among their healthy opposites. And those opposites are: Taking deliberate steps to reduce jet lag, lessen stress, improve on-the-road nutrition, and get regular exercise while traveling. Business travelers who persist with these four counter-measures will find that they work together—in other words, synergistically—to greatly improve their health and fitness, both day by day and over time.

In Chapters One and Two, we took a long look at travel nutrition and exercise. More specifically, we looked at the many dangers of the non-nutritious fare that is typically available to business travelers, versus the food groups that, based on scientific proof, Harvard nutrition researchers recommend as being conducive to good health and optimal well-being.

We also looked at the dangers of sitting for long hours, and getting little or no exercise.

Finally, we saw how Bob, our Health and Fitness Start-up Hero, got started on an exercise routine that he could follow while traveling for his job.

Since we've covered the foundational landscape of travel nutrition and exercise with some thoroughness, let's take a look at jet lag and stress, the two travel-toll inevitabilities we've not yet studied in as much depth. We'll start with the larger category: the role that stress plays in frequent business travel, and how to avoid, reduce, and ultimately eliminate it altogether.

Stress vs. the Relaxation Response

In 1975, Dr. Herbert Benson, a Harvard Medical School cardiologist and researcher, published *The Relaxation Response,* a groundbreaking book that unveiled something of great importance to business travelers.

Dr. Benson had made the discovery that, in the same way that we have a "fight or flight" survival instinct which protects us in situations of sudden, life-threatening danger, we also have a built-in "relaxation response" designed to help us recover from daily stressors which can be illness-inducing after months or years of living in chronically stressful conditions.

Here's another way of looking at these two built-in mechanisms: Fight or flight is the body's protective response to immediate threats to our survival. The relaxation response is the body's protective response to less immediately dangerous but more chronic threats. We rely on both to stay alive—and healthy.

But what is the relaxation response? Perhaps the best way to answer that is with an explanation of what it is not.

When we are chronically stressed, we experience a constant release of the same stress hormones used to prepare our bodies for doing battle with, or running away from, a physical threat. Over time, this constant drip, drip, drip of hormones designed to make us temporarily stronger and faster, actually makes us ill. We may develop immune disorders, or heart disease, or high blood pressure, or even diabetes as a result of experiencing unremitting, chronic, and "ambient-level" stress. In other words, stress we have grown so accustomed to that we no longer perceive it for what it is: a major cause of the gradual degradation of our health and well-being.

Chronic Stress

How does chronic stress have this long-term effect? Our stress hormones (cortisol, ACTH, norepinephrine, epinephrine), which come into play in chronic stress situations, simply wear us out. They do this by amping up our heart rate, blood pressure, respiration, the flow of blood to our muscles, and our metabolic rate, while at the same time shutting down our digestive system and our bodily repair and growth (processes not needed to escape what they perceive as an immediate threat). And these hormones eventually damage our ability to cope with ever-present stress. The next level of degradation is actual disease. And that outcome is the unfortunate result for many.

But it doesn't have to be that way. Our body's innate relaxation response can come to the rescue if we let it.

Here's how it works: When the body transitions into a relaxation response, the release of stress hormones lessens gradually and stops. In its place, we experience an upsurge of the hormones of well-being, particularly endorphins (the same gentle-high hormones that are released after strenuous exercise).

Endorphins counteract all the physical symptoms of stress. They reduce muscle tension, decrease the rate of respiration, slow the heart rate, and lower both blood pressure and metabolism.

At the same time, our brain waves relax when we experience the relaxation response, gradually transitioning from the alert frequencies of beta, to the slower, more tranquil frequencies of alpha, the brain waves that characterize a meditative state.

Inducing the Relaxation Response

Unlike the stress response (in which the body immediately reacts to any perceived threat by triggering a state of hyper-alertness), the relaxation response almost always requires our conscious participation. We need to make a deliberate effort to stimulate it.

So here are the steps that Dr. Benson recommends for stimulating the relaxation response:

Sit comfortably. Close your eyes and breathe deeply, in and out, several times.

Focus on each part of your body to consciously relax your muscles, beginning with your feet and slowly working your way up your legs and torso to your arms, face, and finally, your scalp. Breathe deeply, in and out, while you do so.

Once you have completed your progressive muscle relaxation process, focus on just one thing in order to calm your mind and allow your brain waves to gradually exit beta and enter the slower, more meditative frequencies of alpha.

You could choose to focus on your breath as you breathe in and out, perhaps counting, one, two; one, two. Or you could focus on repeating a single word that is meaningful to you—the word "calm," for instance. Or you might gaze at an object with half-closed eyes A candle flame is often used in meditation, but lighting candles is often discouraged in hotel rooms. You could bring along a photograph of a lake or some other peaceful scene, instead).

Another method for entering the meditative relaxation response is by using visualization. Simply imagine a peaceful environment, as if you were daydreaming or watching a movie inside your mind. Include as many sensory details as you can. Imagine the sounds, smells, sensations (sunlight warming your skin, say) to make your visualization as convincing as possible. These sensory details will help you enter a deeper, more relaxing meditative state.

Your relaxation session can last for ten to twenty minutes, depending upon how stressed you were before you began, and how much time you can devote.

Tools to Stimulate Your Relaxation Response

The above instructions aside, you needn't rely solely on your own internal resources to stimulate your body's relaxation response. Particularly when you're just beginning to use this innate process to protect yourself from stress overload and burnout, you may find it helpful to make use of a number of external relaxation tools to stimulate your relaxation process.

Meditation music. This music genre offers a quick and easy way to shut out the noisy world and enter a peaceful environment of sound. You can find many meditation music examples as both digital downloads and CDs on line (some are even free). In most cases, you can listen to sample tracks online before you invest in music that will transport you to a more tranquil world. Quiet, calming music is inherently therapeutic, offering a no-effort way to release tensions, troubling emotions, and sheer fatigue. The music takes you beyond your business and travel preoccupations, almost in spite of yourself.

Subliminal recordings. These recordings provide soothing music with inaudible relaxation messages that your mind hears, nonetheless, and responds to while you listen. Here are a few examples of inaudible messages imbedded in subliminal recordings: "I am calm and relaxed." "I feel peaceful and tranquil." "My mind is calm." "I am feeling calmer and more relaxed each and every day." It's easy to see how these embedded messages represent a form of hypnosis, since simple, repeated messages tend to entrain your thoughts and change them in positive ways. Like meditation music, subliminal recordings can easily be found online.

Guided imagery recordings. If you feel that you need a little more assistance in getting to a calmer state of mind, guided imagery recordings are often the best choice. They provide an entire visualization journey, a soothing voice that guides you through a peaceful landscape, in which you are helped to experience sounds, sights, and smells as if you were actually visiting a tranquil spot. An experience in total immersion, guided imagery can work wonders in helping you let go of anxiety and stress. You can find excellent examples of guided imagery recordings for relaxation and other positive mind/body states at HealthJourneys.com. You can also find them elsewhere online.

Aromatherapy. Another tool for stress reduction is aromatherapy. At its simplest, this entails inhaling the scent of essential oils (the distilled essence of plants or botanicals). For stress and/or depression, the best choices would be the essential oils of lavender, thyme, and lemon. Smelling one or more of these three essential oils works to lessen stress because the olfactory nerve that controls our sense of smell is physically connected to the brain's limbic system. This part of the brain controls our emotions and also stores the memories associated with certain scents. This explains why the smell of an outdoor fire, say, can instantly bring back enjoyable memories of being eight years old and camping in the woods with your parents and cousins. That scent-memory is preserved in your brain's limbic system. Once the limbic system is stimulated by the scent of one or more of the above essential oils, chemicals are released that induce a state of calm and relaxation. Different essential oils create different results, of course, and there's an essential oil for just about every result you might want. Essential oils are thought to have a bona fide pharmacological effect, one that is instant but subtle. Meanwhile, essential oil bottles are quite small and therefore easy to use, and portable, besides.

Seated chair massage. Many hotels and airports offer seated chair massage for travelers. In case this type of massage is new to you, here's how it works: After straddling a special reverse-back chair while fully clothed, a massage therapist—facing your back, which is turned toward him or her—loosens the tight muscles in your neck, shoulders, arms, hands, and back using vigorous massage. Chair massage also relieves your stress, anxiety, and fatigue at the same time. The reason chair massage is especially useful for you as a business traveler is because you can have a session before or between meetings, since you needn't get undressed and no massage oil is used. Also, good results can be obtained in just ten or fifteen minutes. In fact, it could be worth your while to inquire about the availability of this type of massage at the hotels where you plan to stay, and make your choices of accommodation accordingly.

Cognitive behavior therapy (CBT). When used for stress management, CBT works with the understanding that circumstances do not cause stress as much as our reaction to those circumstances does. During several in-person CBT sessions over the course of a few months. This therapy is very short-term, as it focuses exclusively on a single issue and is not concerned with the past, as other forms of therapy are. A CBT therapist will uncover the negative thoughts that both create stress and make it worse. Then she or he will help you modify your behavior and reframe your thought process, so both become supportive rather than detrimental. CBT has proved successful in providing permanent relief from stress, as well as depression and other common disorders that many frequent business travelers acquire with time.

Exercise. One of the quickest ways to alleviate stress is by metabolizing your stress hormones with a little aerobic exercise. Even if you only walk briskly around the airport—you can stow your carryon luggage and laptop in a locker while you do—or around your hotel parking lot, moving your arms and legs while breathing deeply will soon reduce your level of stress. And, like all the other healthy, anti-stress tools we've mentioned here, there are no negative side effects.

Practice Makes Relaxation Easier and Better

Whatever external tools you choose to use—or not use—in order to reduce your stress and increase your ability to relax, you will probably find that the more you practice the relaxation response, the better you become at inducing it, and the more profound your feeling of relaxation will be. In other words, once you teach your body this new skill, continued practice will make it increasingly easier, and it will eventually become a fully conditioned response requiring little lead time to induce.

The Many FBT Benefits of the Relaxation Response

Here's a nutshell list of all the reasons you might want to develop your relaxation response skill: To decrease pain and muscle tension; to lower blood pressure and stress hormone levels; to lessen travel irritability, simmering anger, nagging anxiety, and sheer fatigue; to improve sleep and decision-making ability; and to increase energy, motivation, and productivity.

Here's one more reason. Stress makes us think in tunnel vision and can even endanger us by keeping us from seeing the larger picture. When we're under stress, we're much more likely to make mistakes and misread situations. We can make bad decisions, damage relationships, and hurt ourselves because we lose perspective on what we're doing.

What business travelers might take away from the dangers of stress and the many methods of de-stressing outlined above is this: With practice, it can be relatively easy to avoid becoming a prisoner of business travel stress. Simply teach yourself to enter a state of physical and mental relaxation, and once you do, you'll be able to leave stressful feelings behind with increasing frequency and success. (In Chapter Four, we'll take a look at what business travelers can do to reduce or even avoid jet lag, a subset of the overall stress syndrome of working on the road.)

Dave, the Health and Fitness Entrepreneur

Our Health and Fitness Entrepreneur, who we'll call Dave, works for a multinational company that pioneered the field of corporate anti-job-stress trainings for employees. As a result, Dave has taken a series of seminars about the causes of job stress, and methods of avoiding the stress sinkhole.

Once Dave adopted many of the strategies he learned in these company seminars, he discovered time that he hadn't noticed before—while waiting in airports, between meetings, and in the evening—when he could sit quietly, focus on his breathing, and feel stress and tension fall away. As an added bonus, Dave found that solutions to difficult work problems often came to him during relaxation sessions, when he was calm enough to access his deeper, alpha-frequency mind.

No Time to Exercise?

But Dave was still troubled by the fact that, when he traveled, he couldn't seem to exercise. Unlike de-stressing with meditation, exercise required a change of clothes and at least thirty minutes, and he never seemed to have that much free time. When Dave was at home, though, he made it to his gym three times a week, and went running in his neighborhood every evening, just to chill out after work.

The reason Dave's lack of on-the-road exercise worried him was because, even though he had only been at this new job for five months, he'd already noticed a decline in his physical health. He tired more easily, and felt generally sluggish and out of sorts when he was traveling, which he did for two or three weeks each month. Even his ability to concentrate seemed impaired. And as if all that wasn't bad enough, he'd also gained about six or seven pounds, so his suits no longer fit the way they used to. This made him feel uncomfortable and ill at ease.

As Dave grew more and more exasperated by the toll his job was taking, he considered quitting and entering another field, even though he was doing well, and was now positioned to move up in his career fairly quickly.

The Travel Fitness Coach Saves the Day

Then Dave heard about the Travel Fitness Coach. On an international flight to the Netherlands, he happened to sit next to another road warrior who lived in his home city. This fellow business traveler told Dave about a coach specializing in travel fitness who helped him find a way to exercise while on the road. As a result, he now felt a hundred times better, since both his physical fatigue and mental fog had disappeared.

Dave was much encouraged by his seatmate's story, and hoped this coach could help him, too. The day after returning from the Netherlands, Dave booked an appointment, signed up, and over the next two weeks, while he was working in his home-city office, met with Steve, his new travel fitness coach, every evening. Steve began by asking Dave to get a complete physical exam, so they'd both know what they were working with, and where they should concentrate their efforts. As it turned out, Dave was in good shape, since he exercised daily when he was at home, but his blood sugar was slightly elevated and he needed to change his diet. Less soda and fast food and more healthy unprocessed food would soon to make a big difference in his blood chemistry, he was told.

After Dave shared the results of his physical, Steve gave him a booklet about healthy meals and food choices, and suggested a good nutritionist who could help him normalize his blood sugar. With better understanding of healthy eating, Dave would be able to eat better while traveling, despite the difficulty of finding healthy food in airports, on airplanes, and in hotel restaurants.

Next, Steve developed exercise routines that were flexible enough to fit Dave's travel schedule. As a result, Dave realized that it wasn't true he had no time to exercise. For a light workout, he didn't have to get changed. He could take brisk walks and stretch or use exercise tubing almost anywhere, at any time. Instead of being a big deal, he began to think of exercise as a continuous pursuit—an all-day, every day habit.

Convincing Clients

Dave even convinced many of his clients to join him in stretching and walking for ten minutes, every hour, during meetings. He did this by explaining that his company was adamant about de-stressing and maintaining excellent health and fitness. It was, in fact, a new stipulation in his employment contract, he explained, and all three areas would be checked twice a year when he received performance reviews. (This last part, while true, was especially useful for excusing himself from unnecessarily late evening meetings, so he could get to bed early enough to exercise before dawn the following morning.)

Dave also cited this aspect of his employee contract as another reason why his global corporation was a superior one to do business with. Since they were willing to invest in the health and fitness of their employees, Dave said, that demonstrated their willingness to be responsible business partners, too.

Not only that, but when potential clients realized that taking brief exercise breaks every hour meant that they all came back to the negotiating table feeling calmer and more relaxed, as well as more able to focus on the work at hand, Dave's point was effectively underscored, and his credibility enhanced. It was definitely a win-win.

The Health and Fitness Entrepreneur Exercise Routine

Dave's travel fitness coach suggested both diet and exercise—in other words, working with a nutritionist, and doing workable exercise routines on the road—as the best way to normalize his blood sugar, lose those extra pounds, and optimize his health and fitness. He also asked Dave to do one more thing: to keep a health and fitness log.

Not an ordinary log, but one kept in two places—on his smart phone, and in a small hardbound notebook about the size of his phone. Steve wanted Dave to email him his log each week for feedback. And he wanted Dave to spend time inputting his notations into a phone app once or twice a week, so Dave would see how well he was doing, and where he might want to do better. Steve also wanted Dave to have all his information in a written form that he could pick up and leaf through, a tangible journal of his health and fitness progress and accomplishments.

Using the template that Steve gave him, Dave would keep daily track of everything he ate and drank, every bit of exercise he did (he also needed to get a pedometer to measure the distances he walked and jogged), and all his relaxation response periods. He also noted whatever insights came to him while exercising or meditating, though he didn't have to share these with Steve, of course.

While it might seem like a lot of work, Steve explained, it was important to keep track, and get encouragement and course-correction, especially in the beginning. Dave could see Steve's point, and he set up his health and fitness log in his smart phone, got several small hardbound notebooks, found a good pedometer online, and purchased exercise tubing with three levels of resistance. He was on his way.

Working with Steve to design a doable, flexible, but excellent exercise routine for the road, Dave decided that he would commit to getting up an hour earlier (something he'd acclimate to while still at home), and he'd get to bed half an hour to an hour earlier to make that early rising time possible. During his extra hour in the morning, Dave would spend his first fifteen minutes doing his relaxation response routine, then a series of limbering up stretches, followed by cardio exercise.

When he was staying in a place that would permit it, Dave would fulfill his cardio requirement by jogging outdoors for about fifteen minutes, or by using a treadmill in the hotel gym. If neither were possible, he'd run up and down the hotel stairs, jog in place, do jumping jacks, or follow the cardio exercise suggestions in the exercise routine

Steve had given him. Any of those options would get his heart rate up.

Then, he'd do post-cardio stretching, followed by strength training exercises (using the multi-layered routine Steve suggested), and end with more stretching. Because Dave had to spend so much time sitting while traveling and in meetings, keeping his muscles well-stretched was especially important.

After that, he'd usually listen to meditation music while focusing on his breathing. Then he'd shower and get on with his day. But Dave's daily exercises didn't end there.

Throughout the day, he'd walk, stretch, use exercise tubing, and maybe even jog a little, in order to keep his body moving and his mind alert—to be at the top of his game. As mentioned earlier, Dave also managed to convert many of his clients to hourly, short exercise routines, because it helped everyone enjoy more productive—and shorter— meetings.

On-the-Road Exercise Program

Here is the four-month program of daily exercises that Steve designed for Dave's on-the-road use. Dave uses it when he wasn't traveling, too, because it stretches, tones, and conditions every part of his body and makes him feel really good. Dave tries to work out every day, but he always takes one day off each week. If he needs to skip a day now and then, that's acceptable—Dave just tries to get back on schedule as soon as he can.

To see how the various exercises and stretches should be done, check my YouTube videos on ReaChannel. YouTube has many other exercise videos as well; another good source is bodybuilding.com.

Month One

Week One: Monday, Wednesday, Friday

Pre-workout stretching	standing toe touches (5 minutes)
Cardio exercise	jumping jacks (5 minutes)
Stretching	neck and hamstring stretches

	(5 minutes each)
Strength training	Starting with the number you can comfortably complete, work up to:
	100 push-ups
	50 burpees
	50 sit-ups
	50 Indian push-ups
	100 body squats
Post-workout stretching	50 upper body twists
Relaxation	10 to 20 minutes

Week One: Tuesday, Thursday, Saturday

Pre-workout stretching	25 windmill stretches
Cardio exercise	jogging in place (5 minutes)
Stretching	25 groin stretches
Strength training	Starting with the number you can comfortably complete, work up to:
	100 desk pulls
	30 pull-ups
	100 crunches
	30 isometric bicep curls
Post-workout stretching	20 lying waist twists
Relaxation	10 to 20 minutes

Week Two: Monday through Friday

Pre-workout stretching	50 leg kicks (25 each leg)
Cardio exercise	jog up and down 3 flights of stairs, twice
Stretching	20 triceps stretches
Strength training	Starting with the number you can comfortably complete, work up to:

	100 push-ups
	30 pull-ups
	100 body squats
	50 Indian push-ups
	100 standing calf raises
	(50 each leg)
Post-workout stretching	oor jamb stretches (3 minutes)
Relaxation	10 to 20 minutes

Week Three: Monday, Tuesday, Friday

Pre-workout stretching	lying thigh stretches
	(1 minute each side)
Cardio exercise	jogging in place (5 minutes)
Stretching	50 toe touches
Strength training	Starting with the number you can comfortably complete, work up to:
	50 jump squats
	50 burpees
	50 Indian push-ups
	100 standing calf raises
	(50 each leg)
Post-workout stretching	25 circular hip stretches
Relaxation	10 to 20 minutes

Week Three: Wednesday, Thursday, Saturday

Pre-workout stretching	seated hip stretch
	(1 minute each side)
Cardio exercise	10 hallway sprints
Stretching	20 groin stretches
Strength training	Starting with the number you can

	comfortably complete, work up to:
	75 pull-ups
	30 isometric biceps curls
	100 bicycle crunches
Post-workout stretching	50 neck stretches,
	50 door jamb stretches
Relaxation	10 to 20 minutes

Week Four: Monday through Friday

Pre-workout stretching	seated thigh stretches (1minute)
Cardio exercise	Stair sprint (3 flights, 3 times)
Stretching	lying hip stretches
	(2 minutes each side)
Strength training	Starting with the number you can
	comfortably complete, work up to:
	15 body squats
	15 lunges
	15 Indian push-ups
	15 pull-ups
	15 dips
	15 sit-ups
Post-workout stretching	50 windmill stretches
Relaxation	10 to 20 minutes

Month Two
Week One: Monday through Friday

Pre-workout stretching	25 standing toe touches
Cardio exercise	jumping jacks (5 minutes)
Stretching	25 circular hip stretches
Strength training	Starting with the number you can
	comfortably complete, work up to:
	20 push-ups

	20 pull-ups
	20 lunges
	20 standing calf raises (10 each leg)
	20 body squats
	20 sit-ups
Post-workout stretching	50 arm spins
Relaxation	10 to 20 minutes

Week Two: Monday, Wednesday, Friday

Pre-workout stretching	50 windmills
Cardio exercise	jogging in place (5 minutes)
Stretching	50 windmills
Strength training	Starting with the number you can comfortably complete, work up to:
	25 body squats
	25 lunges
	25 push-ups
	25 Indian push-ups
Post-workout stretching	lying thigh stretches (3 minutes)
Relaxation	10 to 20 minutes

Week Two: Tuesday, Thursday, Saturday

Pre-workout stretching	10 lat stretches over a desk
Cardio exercise	50 vertical jumps
Stretching	10 seated hamstring stretches
Strength training	Starting with the number you can comfortably complete, work up to:
	10 pull-ups
	20 isometric biceps curls
	50 inverted crunches
Post-workout stretching	lat and bicep stretches (3 minutes each)

Relaxation	10 to 20 minutes

Week Three: Monday through Saturday

Pre-workout stretching	30 leg kicks
Cardio exercise	25 burpees
Stretching	seated groin stretches (2 minutes
Strength training	Starting with the number you can comfortably complete, work up to:
	10 pull-ups
	10 push-ups
	10 lunges
	10 jump squats
	10 bicycle crunches
Post-workout stretching	25 hamstring stretches
Relaxation	10 to 20 minutes

Week Four: Monday, Tuesday, Friday

Pre-workout stretching	25 seated toe touches
Cardio exercise	jog up and down three flights of stairs, 3 times
Stretching	lying hamstring stretches (2 minutes each leg)
Strength training	Starting with the number you can comfortably complete, work up to:
	100 jump squats
	100 lunges
	50 pull-ups
	100 standing calf raises (50 each leg)
Post-workout stretching	10 lateral hamstring stretches
Relaxation	10 to 20 minutes

Week Four: Wednesday, Thursday, Saturday

Pre-workout stretching	25 circular hip stretches
Cardio exercise	10 hallway sprints
Stretching:	5 wide-stance hamstring stretches
Strength training	Starting with the number you can comfortably complete, work up to:
	50 push-ups
	50 Indian push-ups
	50 bent-over triceps extensions
	50 leg raises
Post-workout stretching	seated hip twists (5 minutes)
Relaxation	10 to 20 minutes

Month Three

Week One: Monday through Saturday

Pre-workout stretching	50 windmills
Cardio exercise:	jogging in place (5 minutes)
Stretching	lying hamstring stretch (1 minute each side)
Strength training	continuous vertical jump squats, pull-ups, push-ups (15 minutes)
Post-workout stretching	door jamb stretch (1 minute)
Relaxation	10 to 20 minutes

Week Two: Monday, Wednesday, Friday

Pre-workout stretching	seated groin stretches (3 minutes)
Cardio exercise	jogging in place (5 minutes)
Stretching	hamstring pulls (1 minute)
Strength training	50 pull-ups
	50 sit-ups

Post-workout stretching	25 seated toe touches
Relaxation	10 to 20 minutes

Week One: Tuesday, Thursday, Saturday

Pre-workout stretching	25 arm spins
Cardio exercise	20 burpees
Stretching	20 side leg raises (description; work up to 20
Strength training	Starting with the number you can comfortably complete, work up to:
	50 burpees
	50 Indian push-ups
	50 jump lunges
	50 standing calf raises (25 each leg)
Post-workout stretching	50 windmills
Relaxation	10 to 20 minutes

Week Three: Monday through Friday

Pre-workout stretching	seated leg spread (1 minute
cardio exercise	jogging in place (5 minutes)
Stretching	25 standing toe touches
Strength training	Starting with the number you can comfortably complete, work up to:
	12 pull-ups
	12 chair dips
	12 burpees
	12 squats
	12 lunges
	12 standing calf raises (6 each leg)
	12 leg raises
Post-workout stretching	standing single-leg hamstring stretch (30 seconds each side)

Relaxation	10 to 20 minutes

Week Four: Monday through Saturday

Pre-workout stretching	50 jumping jacks
Cardio exercise	jogging in place (5 minutes)
Stretching	triceps stretches and lat stretches (10 each)
Strength training	Starting with the number you can comfortably complete, work up to: 8 chair dips 8 Indian push-ups 8 pull-ups 8 jump squats 8 lunges 8 standing calf raises (4 each leg) 8 inverted crunches
Post-workout stretching	25 circular hip stretches
Relaxation	10 to 20 minutes

Month Four
Week One: Monday through Friday

Pre-workout stretching	5 bent-over back stretches
Cardio exercise	Jogging in place (5 minutes)
Stretching	seated toe touches (2 minutes)
Strength training	Starting with the number you can comfortably complete, work up to: 10 pull-ups 10 push-ups 10 body squats 10 lunges 10 Indian push-ups 10 sit-ups

Post-workout stretching	25 windmills
Relaxation	10 to 20 minutes

Week Two: Monday, Wednesday, Friday

Pre-workout stretching	15 standing lat stretches
Cardio exercise	25 burpees
Stretching	25 bent-over hamstring stretches
Strength training	Starting with the number you can comfortably complete, work up to:
	50 pull-ups
	50 isometric biceps curls
	50 inverted crunches
Post-workout stretching	25 jumping jacks
Relaxation	10 to 20 minutes

Week Two: Tuesday, Thursday, Saturday

Pre-workout stretching	10 door jamb stretches
Cardio exercise	50 jumping jacks
Stretching	lying thigh stretches (5 minutes)
Strength training	Starting with the number you can comfortably complete, work up to:
	50 push-ups
	50 Indian push-ups
	50 lunges
	50 standing calf raises (25 each leg)
Post-workout stretching	25 circular hip stretches
Relaxation	10 to 20 minutes

Week Three: Monday through Saturday

Pre-workout stretching	20 vertical jumps
Cardio exercise	70 jumping jacks
Stretching	25 standing toe touches

Strength training	Starting with the number you can comfortably complete, work up to:
	15 pull-ups
	15 Indian push-ups
	15 chair dips
	15 lunges
	30 Bulgarian squats (15 each leg)
	15 crunches
	30 standing calf raises (15 each leg)
Post-workout stretching	20 wide-stance body stretches
Relaxation	10 to 20 minutes

Week Four: Monday, Friday, Saturday

Pre-workout stretching	50 lateral leg kicks (25 each leg)
Cardio exercise	10 hallway sprints
Stretching	seated hip stretch (3 minutes)
Strength training	Starting with the number you can comfortably complete, work up to:
	50 pull-ups
	30 isometric biceps curls
	50 lunges
	50 crunches
Post-workout stretching	15 bent-over lat stretches
Relaxation	10 to 20 minutes

Week Four: Tuesday, Wednesday, Thursday

Pre-workout stretching	10 lying hip stretches
Cardio exercise	30 burpees
Stretching	seated lat stretches (3 minutes each side)
Strength training	Starting with the number you can comfortably complete, work up to:

	35 push-ups
	35 chair dips
	35 body squats
	40 standing calf raises (20 each leg)
	35 Indian push-ups
Post-workout stretching	25 circular neck stretches
Relaxation	10 to 20 minutes

Bob Gets Fit

We'll check in with Dave at the end of Chapter Four, once he's had time to work with the program Steve designed for him. But right now, let's see how Bob, our Health and Fitness Start-up Hero, has been doing.

In the year and a half since Bob started working with his trainer, he has progressed to the point where he's nearly ready to graduate to the Health and Fitness Entrepreneur level. His several chronic conditions, which were still at a stage that meant they could be reversed if he took care of himself, have all resolved. He now has a clean bill of health from his physician. And he wants to keep it that way.

He has also lost over half the weight he'd put on, and only has ten pounds to go. Bob is optimistic that he can lose that in another nine months. He has done so well, in fact, that his much-improved self-confidence inspired him to interview for jobs that did not involve travel. He's waiting for a job offer that he's sure will be made in the next week or so. And he couldn't feel better or be happier with his life.

All Bob needed was a workable way to improve his health and fitness, despite his strenuous work and travel schedule. Once he had that, and had put it into practice, he was home free.

Chapter 4: The Health and Fitness CEO: Maintaining Your Edge While Traveling

Have you ever noticed how, when people feel jet-lagged the day after arriving at a spectacular vacation spot, they simply take it in stride? They sleep for part of the next day. They don't push themselves to do anything more strenuous than lie on the beach, or stroll into a restaurant. And, a day or so later, their fatigue, minor headache, and assorted other symptoms are gone. They're ready to do what people look forward to doing on vacation—they're ready to have fun.

The Chronic Jet Lag of FBTs

For frequent business travelers (FBTs), though, the jet lag that they experience is not the same thing at all. Far more than a minor inconvenience, it's a major detriment to their health, mental well-being, and job performance.

Why the big difference between vacation-traveler jet lag and the jet lag that assails frequent business travelers? It's largely because business travelers traverse multiple time zones during half to two-thirds of every month. For them, jet lag is a "repetitive stress injury." That is, it happens again and again. Every time a frequent business traveler flies across the country, or flies to another continent, and every time he flies back across the country, or to his home continent, jet lag happens, and continues to happen multiple times—month, after month, after month.

Frequent business travelers aren't suffering from the relatively mild-mannered jet lag that vacation travelers sometimes experience.

No. What they have is chronic jet lag, a compounded condition because it occurs repetitively, and with little relief between episodes. So let's look at what jet lag—or circadian dysrhythmia—really is, and why it occurs.

The Science of Jet Lag

Fundamentally, the symptoms of jet lag are the result of a misalignment between a traveler's internal circadian clock (the physiological mechanism that tells the body when to wake up each day and when to go to sleep each night), and the hours of daylight and darkness in a new location, one that's multiple time zones away from their home time zone.

Here's how it works: When daylight enters the retinas at the back of a traveler's eyes, it travels through the optic nerve and signals the brain's hypothalamus that it's time to be awake. As a result, a traveler's body inhibits melatonin, the hormone that assists sleep, and releases cortisol, the hormone that stimulates wakefulness.

But when daylight turns to darkness, the hypothalamus tells the pineal gland, a small endocrine gland at the center of the traveler's brain, to again release an increasing amount of melatonin, thus stimulating the process of preparing for sleep by calming and quieting the organs and lowering the body temperature. This is what happens daily, and the body gets used to the same hours for sleeping and waking each day, used to its particular circadian rhythm.

When a business traveler flies from New York to Los Angeles, however, he steps out of his normal rhythm. He "loses" three hours, traveling backward in time as he crosses all the time zones inside the borders of the United States.

If he leaves New York at 10:00 a.m., say, and his nonstop flight takes six and a half hours, he arrives in Los Angeles at 1:30 p.m., California time, while the time at his east coast departure location will be 4:30 p.m.. As a result, his body would expect to get ready for sleep in six or seven hours, according to its usual circadian rhythm. But in

Los Angeles, his body will have to wait nine or ten hours before sleep. The difference between those two light-dark cycles can and often do create the symptoms of jet lag.

Of course, the difference between six and nine hours (or seven and ten hours) is not extreme; only four time zones were involved :Eastern, Central, Mountain, and Pacific. But when business travelers fly between continents, they cross ten or more time zones and must cross make the adjustment from their home time zone to their business time zone. That will almost certainly lead to jet lag.

The Many Symptoms of Jet Lag

Circadian dysrhythmia affects every traveler differently, as you might expect, but its severity has to do with the total number of time zones crossed, and whether the flight was from west to east (most difficult), or from east to west (not as difficult).

That said, research conducted by British Airways has shown that jet lag and its attendant sleep loss can impair communication skills by 30 percent; diminish memory by 20 percent; and compromise decision-making ability by 50 percent.

For frequent business travelers, such percentages add up to a significant impairment of their executive skills. And that can't help but reduce their effectiveness for their companies, which could, in turn, lead to significant financial losses. So, it's in the best interest of companies with frequent business travelers to help them mitigate their jet lag, as we'll see when we discuss the anti-jet lag strategies that Ed, our Health and Fitness CEO, employs.

But first, let's take a look at some of the actual symptoms of jet lag:

Daytime Fatigue

Fatigue is the most common jet lag symptom, and 90 percent of all travelers experience daytime tiredness and sleepiness as a result of being out of sync with the time zone they've just flown to for business. Many also experience headaches due to travel stress and anxiety (catching flights on time, getting through security), and due also to low humidity and low cabin pressure (leading to reduced oxygen in the bloodstream) that is common on jetliners.

Poor Concentration and Temporary Memory Loss

After traversing multiple time zones, it's almost as if a traveler's brain synapses lose their ability to function. More than two-thirds of all travelers experience:

• Inability to think clearly
• Inability to concentrate their attention and focus
• Inability to remember things they know well under normal circumstances
• Inability to write in a coherent manner

In extreme cases, a traveler may experience temporary amnesia of a limited type, or less commonly, of a more far-reaching type. As a subset of brain dysfunction, some travelers also find themselves feeling irritable and even angry. In other words, their moods alter in a negative way as a result of jet lag.

Disorientation

A great many business travelers experience disorientation, having difficulty remembering where they are, and feeling confused if they waken in the middle of the night and find themselves in strange surroundings.

Slowed Reflexes

Just as mental processes seem scrambled and dysfunctional when a traveler is suffering from jet lag, physical processes are affected, as well, with some reporting greatly slowed-down reflexes (so driving a rental car could prove dangerous).

Insomnia

Along with daytime fatigue, an inability to sleep is extremely common among jet-lag sufferers. And once sleep arrives, it is often punctuated by frequent episodes of waking up, probably because deep sleep is typically impossible with the onset of jet lag.

Gastrointestinal Difficulties
Half of all travelers experience various forms of digestive disruption, including no appetite, feelings of hunger at strange hours, heartburn, and constipation. All the body's functions are out of sync, and the digestive tract is no exception.

The Catch-22 of Frequent Business Travel
It's ironic, but frequent business travelers are prone to develop a variety of chronic illnesses (discussed in earlier chapters), and those illnesses tend to make the symptoms of jet lag not only worse, they could worsen to a degree that results in a medical emergency.

This doesn't seem fair. That a frequent business traveler may have forfeited his health in order to do his job, and may also suffer a severe reaction to jet lag because of chronic illnesses resulting from that job, seems like a particularly pernicious Catch-22 situation.

On the other hand, experiencing a health crisis could just be a wake-up call. It might be the incentive needed to either pay greater attention to your health and fitness on the road, or switch to a less taxing job, at least temporarily, in order to focus on repairing your health.

For the frequent business traveler who isn't at a health crisis point, though, there are many ways to handle the added stress of jet lag. We'll look at some of them, below.

How NASA Dispels Astronaut Jet Lag
American astronauts frequently travel among international space agencies in Europe, Japan, and Russia, so NASA has developed effective methods for alleviating jet lag. The NASA methods work two to three times faster than is considered average for circadian dysrhythmia recovery.

In part, these methods work so quickly because they are tailored to each astronaut's precise physiological parameters. But the three basic principles that NASA employs can still prove helpful in designing your own methods for mitigating and even preventing jet lag.

The first travel factor that NASA makes use of when counteracting jet lag is the direction of travel, whether an astronaut is flying east or west across multiple time zones. If flying east, prior to a scheduled flight, an astronaut will be encouraged to advance his body clock (circadian rhythm) to more closely match his destination's time zone. He'll do this by going to bed earlier and waking up earlier, in small increments of half an hour per day, for a week or so. And while it won't be possible to advance an astronaut's body clock so much that it's completely in sync with his destination's time zone, even a partial advance will reduce the symptoms of jet lag. (If he's flying west, on the other hand, the goal would be the reverse—to delay his body clock by going to bed later and waking up later.)

The second travel factor that NASA makes use of is what speeds recovery from jet lag significantly, and it involves something very simple: controlling an astronaut's exposure to light. If flying east, not only will an astronaut need to go to sleep earlier and wake up earlier, he will need to also be exposed to light earlier (whether sunlight or artificial light). If flying west, light exposure should occur in the early evening to delay the body clock mechanism that prepares an astronaut for sleep. Another trick NASA uses is giving sunglasses to its astronauts in order to minimize light exposure, when such exposure would reset their body clocks for the wrong direction.

Finally, the time of the flight (morning, afternoon, night) is the third travel element that NASA takes into consideration in helping its astronauts reduce their potential jet lag. Depending upon whether an astronaut will arrive at his destination at night or in broad daylight, he will be encouraged to either sleep on the plane, or to get as much light on his flight as possible, in order to mimic what people in his new time zone are experiencing. On a night flight, for instance, he might sleep through the flight with the aid of an eye mask and ear plugs (and perhaps a dose of valerian, a herbal relaxer and gentle sleep-inducer with no side effects), and arrive at an early morning hour when his destination city is just waking up, as he, too, will then be.

Once he arrives, NASA will have cautioned him to avoid alcohol and heavy, spicy meals in the evening before bedtime, as alcohol can lead to disturbed sleep patterns, and a heavy meal can lead to wakefulness. In general, carbohydrates, as found in vegetables and grain dishes, are relaxing and sleep-inducing, while heavy proteins like meat and poultry, and even some fish, will keep a traveler awake at night.

Additional Ways to Mitigate Jet Lag

In addition to trying to follow the NASA method, look into other ways to keep jet lag to a minimum.

Drink Lots of Water

Jetliner cabins not only force passengers to breathe partially recycled air for many hours, the air they breathe is also extremely dry, with an average of just 20 percent humidity. As a result, drinking lots of water can offset a tendency to become dehydrated, as well as to develop a resultant headache. A *New England Journal of Medicine* study reported that fatigue, muscle pain, headaches, and malaise were common on long flights. The cause is the low cabin pressure on jetliners. That low pressure leads to a 4 percent reduction in the oxygen circulated by a traveler's bloodstream; in other words, there is also a certain amount of oxygen "starvation" which contributes to the symptoms cited above.

Stand Up, Stretch, Move Around

Sitting for long hours isn't good for anyone, but it's especially bad for travelers sitting in cramped quarters with few options for even minimal physical exercise. For some people, sitting for much of a twenty-hour flight can lead to swelling, or edema, in the legs and feet. There is also the danger of blood clot formation in the legs (known as deep vein thrombosis, and discussed earlier). But for those in relatively good health, it is still important to stretch periodically, walk up and down the aisles, and move around as much as possible, particularly on long flights. Such movement will help to offset the severity of jet lag.

Block Out Light Noise

If you are planning to sleep on your flight, because that will help you synchronize with the time zone of your destination, be sure to use an eye mask and ear plugs to block out light and reduce ambient noise. Once you've arrived and are ready to go to bed in your hotel room, do the same thing, so you won't be disturbed in your new environment. Another way to ensure a good night's sleep in a different time zone is to take a hot bath before bed. It will help relax your muscles and ease your physical fatigue and stress.

Arrive Several Days Early

When you have important meetings to attend, it's wise to arrive at your destination a few days early, in order to have the time you need to adjust to the new time zone. You want to be sure that your mental faculties and physical functions have returned to a relatively normal state.

And while the expense of adding days to your trip may be something your company balks at, the lost business from a botched high-level meeting—botched because of jet lag—could cost far more. You need to be in top form to do well in meetings, and arriving early will help you get there more quickly.

Ed, Our Health and Fitness CEO

Ed, our Health and Fitness CEO, is a good example of an executive whose value to his company has given him the leverage to negotiate a beneficial frequent travel agreement— beneficial to Ed and his company, both.

But before we look at the contract that Ed negotiated, let's see how he arrived at this particular juncture in his career. To do that, we'll need to look back in time—three decades back.

When Ed was in elementary school, his family moved every few years (his father was an Air Force officer who later became a military consultant), so Ed and his older sister and brother were always the new kids at school, which sometimes made them the target of teasing, and worse.

In Ed's case, though, there was an added burden. From the second grade through the sixth, he was a chubby kid, which not only made the teasing especially painful, it meant that few kids wanted to risk their social status by befriending him. So even though Ed's brother and sister gradually made friends and got invited to birthday parties and other events, he spent his time after school and on weekends by himself. His worried parents tried to help their youngest child fit in. But their efforts largely failed.

Then, during the summer before Ed's seventh grade year—his first year in junior high— his family prepared to move again. Ed decided to use that summer to make a big change in his appearance before entering yet another new school in the fall. He convinced his parents to let him attend a hiking and camping summer camp. And, for two months, plus an additional two weeks when he helped close the camp up for the winter, Ed was outdoors, engaged in strenuous activities all day, every day, while consuming nutritious meals and no junk food snacks.

The change was miraculous. When Ed got home at the end of that summer, his family hardly recognized him. Their chubby little boy was not only baby-fat-free, he had grown several inches taller, and could display a set of biceps that any twelve-year-old would be proud of.

But Ed wasn't just physically changed. His new-found confidence in his appearance gave him the inner strength to reach out to boys his own age. And, after befriending all the kids at the end of his new block, Ed finally discovered what it was like to be popular and have a group of friends.

When school started a few weeks later, Ed signed up for swimming classes and later convinced his junior high phys ed teacher to give weight-training classes to him and a small group of his classmates. Ed's seventh grade year was a big turning point in his life. He left behind the loneliness and misery of his elementary school years. And he never wanted to go back there again.

As you might imagine, working at being physically fit became a lifelong preoccupation, something as essential to his self-esteem as it was to his social success. Each step of his school journey, as Ed went through high school, college, and business school, he made time for fitness and healthy meals (something he'd learned a lot about, along the way) as the foundation of his daily life.

If we fast-forward another decade or so to Ed's corporate career, we can see that he has cultivated a reputation among his business peers for being unusually physically fit, and unusually successful as a business negotiator. If a deal is impossible, Ed can make it possible.

What he would tell you, though, is that his fitness and his negotiation skills are very much related. In fact, when Ed's pharmaceutical company first offered him a job traveling internationally for up to two-thirds of every month, he made it clear that he would only take the position if his company supported him in maintaining his health and fitness while doing the job. Since his company realized how valuable Ed was to their international plans, they agreed.

So Ed took several trial flights, during which he discovered that arriving two days prior to his scheduled meetings was ideal. And that it was also optimal to stay in a hub locale and travel short distances to meet with representatives of five or six companies, say, during the day, and return to his hub hotel, each night. And that if he stayed two days after his meetings were over, he could reset his body clock before the trip home and avoid jet lag. During those reset days, he would tie up any loose ends and generally finalize the results of all his meetings, so nothing would be lost, as far as his company was concerned.

But that wasn't all that Ed learned on his trial flights; more than mere jet lag was at stake. He also needed to ensure his physical and mental fitness during a grueling travel schedule. So he asked his company for special accommodations that would help him to do just that.

Specifically, Ed asked for a hotel room with a kitchenette (refrigerator, stove, oven, dishes, utensils, pots, and pans), so he could buy groceries and make healthy meals and snacks. He also asked his company to book him into hotels with an on-site gym facility and swimming pool, so he could do his daily workout routine without wasting time traveling to a local gym.

Because Ed was essential to his company's international expansion plans, and because he was so persuasive about the potential for immediate and long-term financial losses—as well as lost business opportunities—due to jet-lag impairment, Ed's company agreed to his travel and accommodation requests as part of his benefits package. They wrote both into his contract.

Maintain Your Health and Fitness without Much Leverage

Of course, not everyone is so well-positioned that they can ask for, and get, healthy nutrition and fitness maintenance accommodations, especially when just starting out. Ed had been with his company for nearly a decade, during which time he'd created a stellar track record.

On the other hand, research on the physical cost of frequent business travel is compelling. So any responsible company should be willing to help its frequent business travelers stay healthy on the road, if only because it's far more expensive to replace a valued employee after he develops health issues than it is to help him stay healthy in the first place.

But if we set aside, for the moment, what a company can do to help its traveling executives, there is still a great deal that the frequent business traveler can do himself to maintain and perhaps improve his health on the road. He can take many of the steps that Ed does. Like Ed, you can partially reset your body clock to your destination's time zone before every flight; pack lots of healthy snacks for the plane, the airport, and travel within the destination country; make time to exercise each day, preferably in the morning and/or the evening, as well as throughout the day on meeting breaks.

Packing Healthy Snacks

Okay, you may be thinking, I could probably do all that. But what are those healthy snacks that Ed packs, and what does he do with that kitchenette?

Ed packs snacks that are filling enough to stave off hunger, and substantial enough to nourish his body until his next real meal, since he knows that flight delays and missed connections are all but inevitable when traveling internationally.

Using resealable, sandwich-size bags, Ed fills about a dozen with organic dried fruit (the nonorganic variety is preserved with sulfur dioxide, which isn't healthy), and organic nuts that are mostly roasted but unsalted. His dried fruit snacks might include raisins, apricots, cranberries, and cherries. And the nuts he packs might include almonds, cashews, walnuts, and sunflower seeds.

Next, Ed fills five or so bags with fat-free granola, and four or so bags with carrot and celery sticks. He takes along hummus (wrapped up in small packets of plastic wrap that are then double-stored in baggies) as a dip for the vegetables. After that, he makes several sandwiches of organic peanut butter and fruit-juice-sweetened jam on whole grain bread (or sesame tahini and honey on whole grain), and cuts each sandwich into four smaller sandwiches (easier to eat on the run), and packs those, too, in baggies. Sometimes, he'll take along a few hard-boiled eggs and use the hummus as a dip, or pack a little salt and pepper. And he always takes along well-washed organic grapes and apples.

With a total of thirty or so small sandwich bags, Ed has found that storing them in square plastic food containers in the bottom of his carry-on bag is the best way to keep them organized and safe, and that also makes them easy for security to inspect. Ed takes along three empty aluminum water bottles, too, which he fills with spring water after going through security (no liquids are allowed through the inspection process).

Packing healthy snacks for the many unknowns of international travel gives Ed peace of mind, so he can focus on preparing for his meetings, staying relaxed, and enjoying whatever he's doing in the moment. And, as you might expect, Ed has found many opportunities to share his snacks with fellow business travelers, while introducing them to the idea of avoiding unhealthy airport and airline food.

But isn't that a lot of trouble, packing all those snacks? Actually, it isn't. Ed spends less than an hour getting his snack supply ready (it's mostly "fill and seal," after all), and being prepared in this way saves him from compromising his health by eating faux food while traveling, or even going hungry when nothing is available during, let's say, an unexpected tarmac wait.

The other reason it's imminently worth it is because having a meal backup means Ed will never have to worry about where he's going to get something to eat, either very early in the morning or very late at night. This simple precautionary measure offers big rewards in terms of reducing one source of travel anxiety, as any frequent business traveler will understand.

About That Kitchenette . . .

Okay, so what about Ed's hotel kitchenette? What does he use it for?

To understand how Ed uses his business destination kitchen, you need to know that he's not a fan of drinks and dinner with prospects and clients in the evening. Ed has discovered that, while there is a certain amount of social bonding that goes on during these occasions, very little real business gets done. So he steers his meeting partners toward early morning meetings that usually end before lunchtime as the best use of their mutual time. And if it turns out that more time is needed, Ed lobbies for meeting again the next morning, rather than continuing on into the afternoon and evening hours. He doesn't always succeed in getting his preferred schedule, but often enough, people see the wisdom of his morning meetings and go along.

Of course, Ed has a hidden health agenda. He wants to get his in-person meetings out of the way in the early morning so he can get back to his hub hotel, make a healthy lunch for himself, and then do emails, phone calls, and paperwork during the afternoon hours. Then, toward the end of the day, and before making himself dinner, Ed will complete another workout (a companion session to his workout in the morning) and go swimming to relax and rejuvenate.

Even though Ed can't always follow his preferred schedule, that fact never stops him from returning to his routine on the next trip, and convincing his meeting partners that early morning sessions are the best use of everyone's time.

And Ed's kitchenette? He uses his kitchen accommodation to make himself breakfast (whole grain hot cereal with fruit and whole grain toast with tahini); to make lunch and snacks (salads, bean and vegetable soups, green smoothies, crunchy vegetables with bean dip); and to make dinner (stir-fried vegetables with tofu or tempeh and sometimes, fish; vegetarian chili; baked vegetable casseroles).

Ed's options are endless, and limited only by the organic produce he can find in the country he's visiting. If he knows that it will be hard to get what he needs, Ed may send himself a package of food by air courier before leaving; he feels the expense is more than worth it, as healthy food is what helps him stay at the top of his game.

The Gym and the Pool?

What about the other part of Ed's health and fitness job contract, the in-hotel gym and swimming pool?

While it's certainly true that Ed can't always get all the daily exercise he prefers, he schedules his days so he can go to bed early and get up early, and after a morning meditation (to relax and "download" business insights from his meditating mind), he goes to the hotel gym for a complete workout that takes about half an hour.

Once his morning meetings are over, Ed returns to his hotel to make lunch for himself, and spends the afternoon working in his room. Before dinner, he does a second workout in the gym and then hits the pool for a relaxation swim, one that helps to drain away all his accumulated stress and tension.

After a healthy dinner, he might take a walk if the grounds or area around his hotel are scenic, but he always gets to bed early so he can get up early and have the time he needs for his morning workout.

Why FBTs Are Road Athletes

Frequent business travelers are athletes in disguise. They are professional travelers, a strenuous sport. And so they need to cultivate, build, and maintain their health and fitness for their FBT sport. in the same way that any athlete must cultivate, build, and maintain the health and fitness he needs to perform: through planning, training, and constant practice.

Like Ed, business travelers with a high level of health and fitness have found doable ways of overcoming jet lag; releasing constant stress; compensating for a scarcity of healthy meal options; and working around the travel reality of having little or no time for daily exercise.

The Health and Fitness CEO Four-Month Exercise Plan

Here is a four-month routine appropriate for those who, like Ed, have been working out for many years, have no chronic conditions, and can pace themselves. This routine lets your pace yourself, not overdoing your exercise, but giving your body the kind of workout it needs to be healthy.

You can adjust the time period for each exercise according to the amount of time you have, and according to your level of fitness. It's far better to do a variety of exercises for a shorter period of time than it is to do no exercise, or to do too much.

Build slowly, even if you are in excellent shape. Remember that travel takes a toll, even with the best precautions. Allow your body to recover, especially during the first few days in a new location. The program below is designed to be done six out of seven days a week. Always take one day off!

I have posted many videos on YouTube showing how to do the various exercises in this plan. Search for them under the ReaShape channel. You can also search YouTube for videos posted by many other trainers or check bodybuilding.com for videos.

Month One
Week One: Monday, Wednesday, Friday

Pre-workout stretching	lying down hamstring stretch (1 minute each side)
Cardio exercise	30 squat thrusts
Stretching	standing body twist (3 minutes)
Strength training	Starting with the number you can comfortably complete, work up to 5 sets of 20 each, or:
	100 pull-ups
	100 isometric biceps curls
	100 lunges
	100 leg raises
Post-workout stretching	seated groin stretch (3 minutes)
Relaxation	10 to 20 minutes

Week One: Tuesday, Thursday, Saturday

Pre-workout stretching	standing hamstring and lat stretches (3 minutes each)
Cardio exercise	burpees (10 minutes)
Stretching	windmill stretches (5 minutes)
Strength training	Starting with the number you can comfortably complete, work up to 5 sets of 20 each, or:
	100 dips
	100 Indian push-ups
	100 body squats
	100 calf raises (50 each leg)
	100 upside-down shoulder presses

	100 neck raises
Post-workout stretching	chest fly stretches (2 minutes)
Relaxation	10 to 20 minutes

Week Two: Monday, Wednesday, Friday

Pre-workout stretching	wide-stance body stretch (3 minutes)
Cardio exercise	run up and down 3 flights of stairs 5 times (start with a comfortable number of flights, then build up)
Strength training	Starting with the number you can comfortably complete, work up to 10 sets of 10 each, or:
	100 push-ups
	100 dips
	100 Indian push-ups
	100 body squats
	100 upside-down shoulder presses
Post-workout stretching	seated thigh stretch (3 minutes)
Relaxation	10 to 20 minutes

Week Two: Tuesday, Thursday, Saturday

Pre-workout stretching	calf stretch and lat stretch (3 minutes each)
Cardio exercise	20 hallway sprints
Stretching	standing circular stretch (1 minute)
Strength training	Starting with the number you can comfortably complete, work up to 15 sets of 10 each, or:
	150 pull-ups
	150 lunges
	150 standing calf raises (75 each leg)

	150 crunches
Post-workout stretching	30 side-to-side hamstring and lat stretches
Relaxation	10 to 20 minutes

Week Three: Monday, Thursday, Friday

Pre-workout stretching	50 toe touch stretches
Cardio exercise	burpees and squat thrusts (3 minutes each)
Stretching	door jamb stretches (3 minutes)
Strength training	Starting with the number you can comfortably complete, work up to: 100 push-ups 70 Indian push-ups 50 upside-down shoulder presses
Post-workout stretching	arm spins (3 minutes)
Relaxation	10 to 20 minutes

Week Three: Tuesday, Wednesday, Saturday

Pre-workout stretching	neck stretches (3 minutes)
Cardio exercise	jog in place (3 minutes)
Stretching	50 windmills
Strength training	Starting with the number you can comfortably complete, work up to: 100 pull-ups 100 lunges 50 body squats 50 calf raises (25 each leg) 50 leg raises 50 head raises
Post-workout stretching	biceps and hamstring stretches 1(3 minutes each)

Relaxation	10 to 20 minutes

Week Four: Monday, Tuesday, Saturday

Pre-workout stretching	50 windmills
Cardio exercise	vertical jumps (3 minutes)
Stretching	25 toe touch kicks (25 each leg)
Strength training	Starting with the number you can comfortably complete, work up to:
	100 Indian push-ups
	50 upside-down shoulder presses
	50 bent-over triceps extensions
	50 standing calf raises (25 each leg)
Post-workout stretching	seated toe touches (3 minutes)
Relaxation	10 to 20 minutes

Week Four: Wednesday, Thursday, Friday

Pre-workout stretching	25 cross-leg toe touches
Cardio exercise	squat thrusts (5 minutes)
Stretching	25 cross-leg toe touches
Strength training	Starting with the number you can comfortably complete, work up to:
	100 jump squats
	50 lunges
	100 pull-ups
	30 isometric biceps curls
	100 bicycle crunches
Post-workout stretching	seated toe touches (3 minutes)
Relaxation	10 to 20 minutes

Month Two

Week One: Monday, Wednesday, Friday

Pre-workout stretching	25 cross leg toe touches
Cardio exercise	40 jump squats
Stretching	lying bent-over hamstring stretch (3 minutes)
Strength training	Starting with the number you can comfortably complete, work up to:
	75 body squats
	50 lunges
	75 Indian push-ups
	50 dips
Post-workout stretching	standing hamstring and triceps stretches (3 minutes each)
Relaxation	10 to 20 minutes

Week Two: Monday, Wednesday, Friday

Pre-workout stretching	wide-stance bent-over hamstring stretch (1 minute)
Cardio exercise	vertical jumps (2 minutes)
Stretching	bent-over lat stretches (2 minutes)
Strength training	Starting with the number you can comfortably complete, work up to:
	50 body squats
	30 lunges
	50 push-ups
	50 Indian push-ups
Post-workout stretching	circular hip stretch (2 minutes)
Relaxation	10 to 20 minutes

Week Two: Tuesday, Thursday, Saturday

Pre-workout stretching	bent-over hamstring stretch (2 minutes)

Cardio exercise	20 hallway sprints
Stretching	seated hamstring stretch (2 minutes)
Strength training	plank (3 minutes)
Post-workout stretching	lying hamstring stretch (1 minute each side)
Relaxation	10 to 20 minutes

Week Three: Monday, Tuesday, Wednesday

Pre-workout stretching	standing wide-stance circular upper body stretch (3 minutes)
Cardio exercise	jogging in place (5 minutes)
Stretching	wide-stance bent-over lower back and hamstring stretches (3 minutes each)
Strength training	Starting with the number you can comfortably complete, work up to 7 sets, 12 repetitions, or:
	84 push-ups
	84 dips
	84 Bulgarian squats
	84 lunges
	84 upside-down shoulder presses
Post-workout stretching	wide-stance seated stretches (3 minutes)
Relaxation	10 to 20 minutes

Week Three: Thursday, Friday, Saturday

Pre-workout stretching	50 standing windmills
Cardio exercise	squat thrusts (2 minutes)
Stretching	hamstring stretches (3 minutes each leg)
Strength training	Starting with the number you can comfortably complete, work up to 7 sets, 12 repetitions, or:

	84 pull-ups
	84 chin-ups
	84 isometric biceps curls
	84 sit-ups
	84 calf raises (42 each leg)
Post-workout stretching	lying hamstring stretch (3 minutes each side)
Relaxation	10 to 20 minutes

Week Four: Monday, Wednesday, Thursday

Pre-workout stretching	arm swings (1 minute)
Cardio exercise	burpees and vertical jumps (2 minutes each)
Stretching	wide-stance opposite toe touches (3 minutes) Strength training Starting with the number you can comfortably complete, work up to 10 sets, 10 repetitions, or:
	100 body squats
	100 pull-ups
	100 dips
	100 leg raises
Post-workout stretching	50 jumping jacks
Relaxation	10 to 20 minutes

Week Four: Tuesday, Friday, Saturday

Pre-workout stretching	50 windmills
Cardio exercise	squat thrusts (10 minutes)
Stretching	door jamb lat stretches (3 minutes)
Strength training	Starting with the number you can comfortably complete, work up to 10 sets, 10 repetitions, or:

	100 Indian push-ups
	100 upside-down push-ups
	100 standing calf raises (50 each leg)
	100 push-ups
Post-workout stretching	lying thigh stretches (3 minutes)
Relaxation	10 to 20 minutes

Month Three
Week One: Monday, Wednesday, Friday

Pre-workout stretching	crab stretch (2 minutes)
Cardio exercise	jogging in place (2 minutes)
Stretching	15 lying V-ups
Strength training	Starting with the number you can comfortably complete, work up to 5 sets, 15 repetitions, or:
	75 pull-ups
	75 crunches
	80 standing calf raises (40 each leg)
Post-workout stretching	bent-over lat stretch (3 minutes)
Relaxation	10 to 20 minutes

Week One: Tuesday, Thursday, Saturday

Pre-workout stretching	chest fly stretches (2 minutes)
Cardio exercise (2 minutes each)	vertical jumps and burpees
Stretching	50 jumping jacks
Strength training	Starting with the number you can comfortably complete, work up to 5 sets, 20 repetitions, or:
	100 push-ups
	100 dips
	25 upside-down shoulder presses

	25 Indian push-ups
Post-workout stretching	50 windmills
Relaxation	10 to 20 minutes

Week Two: Monday, Friday, Saturday

Pre-workout stretching	seated hamstring stretches (3 minutes)
Cardio exercise	jog up and down 3 flights of stairs, 3 times
Stretching	seated hamstring stretches (3 minutes)
Strength training	Starting with the number you can comfortably complete, work up to:
	200 body squats
	175 push-ups
	250 standing calf raises (125 each leg)
	100 crunches
Post-workout stretching	side-to-side leg stretches (3 minutes)
Relaxation	10 to 20 minutes

Week Two: Tuesday, Wednesday, Thursday

Pre-workout stretching	30 lateral leg kicks
Cardio exercise	20 hallway sprints
Stretching	25 circular neck stretches
Strength training	Starting with the number you can comfortably complete, work up to:
	30 upside-down shoulder presses
	40 pull-ups
	35 dips
	25 lunges
Post-workout stretching	30 toe touches
Relaxation	10 to 20 minutes

Week Three: Monday, Tuesday, Thursday

Pre-workout stretching	50 windmills
Cardio exercise	burpees (5 minutes)
Stretching	seated hamstring stretches (3 minutes)
Strength training	Starting with the number you can comfortably complete, work up to:
	100 dips
	75 lunges
	75 leg raises
	30 upside-down shoulder presses
Post-workout stretching	50 jumping jacks
Relaxation	10 to 20 minutes

Week Three: Wednesday, Friday, Saturday

Pre-workout stretching	lying bent-over hamstring stretch (3 minutes)
Cardio exercise	burpees, squat thrusts, jogging in place (2 minutes each)
Stretching	50 windmills
Strength training	Starting with the number you can comfortably complete, work up to:
	100 push-ups
	50 Indian push-ups
	75 body squats
	100 calf raises (50 each leg)
Post-workout stretching	seated thigh stretches (2 minutes)
Relaxation	10 to 20 minutes

Week Four: Monday, Wednesday, Friday

Pre-workout stretching	lat stretches (3 minutes)
Cardio exercise	50 body squats

Stretching:	seated thigh stretches (2 minutes)
Strength training	Starting with the number you can comfortably complete, work up to:
	75 body squats
	30 lunges
	40 upside-down shoulder presses
	75 bicycle crunches
Post-workout stretching	standing hamstring stretch (3 minutes)
Relaxation	10 to 20 minutes

Week Four: Tuesday, Thursday, Saturday

Pre-workout stretching	standing single leg stretch (2 minutes each leg)
Cardio exercise	30 hallway sprints
Stretching	door jamb stretches (3 minutes)
Strength training	Starting with the number you can comfortably complete, work up to:
	50 dips
	50 Indian push-ups
	50 pull-ups
	50 standing calf raises (25 each leg)
Post-workout stretching	lying back stretch (3 minutes)
Relaxation	10 to 20 minutes

Month Four

Week One: Monday, Friday, Saturday

Pre-workout stretching	standing triceps and hamstring stretches (3 minutes each)
Cardio exercise	20 hallway sprints
Stretching	lying hamstring stretch (3 minutes)
Strength training	Starting with the number you can comfortably complete, work up to:

	100 jump squats
	100 Indian push-ups
Post-workout stretching	
Relaxation	10 to 20 minutes

Week One: Tuesday, Wednesday, Thursday

Pre-workout stretching	50 windmills with neck turns
Cardio exercise	squat thrusts and burpees (2 minutes each)
Stretching	50 lateral leg kicks
Strength training	Starting with the number you can comfortably complete, work up to:
	100 pull-ups
	30 upside-down shoulder presses
Post-workout stretching	50 jumping jacks
Relaxation	10 to 20 minutes

Week Two: Monday, Wednesday, Friday

Pre-workout stretching	arm spins (3 minutes)
Cardio exercise	50 burpees
Stretching	25 cross-leg touches
Strength training	Starting with the number you can comfortably complete, work up to 5 sets, 15 repetitions, or:
	75 lunges
	75 upside-down shoulder presses
	75 dips
	80 standing calf raises (40 each leg)
Post-workout stretching	25 jumping jacks
Relaxation	10 to 20 minutes

Week Two: Tuesday, Thursday, Saturday

Pre-workout stretching	30 windmills
Cardio exercise	jog up and down 3 flights of stairs, 3 times
Stretching	lying thigh stretches (3 minutes)
Strength training	Starting with the number you can comfortably complete, work up to 5 sets, 15 repetitions, or:
	75 pull-ups
	75 body squats
	75 crunches
	75 Indian push-ups
Post-workout stretching	lying thigh stretches (3 minutes)
Relaxation	10 to 20 minutes

Week Three: Monday, Tuesday, Wednesday

Pre-workout stretching	door jamb stretches (3 minutes)
Cardio exercise	stair jog (5 minutes)
Stretching	25 leg kicks
Strength training	Starting with the number you can comfortably complete, work up to:
	75 push-ups
	50 Indian push-ups
	40 upside-down shoulder presses
	75 bicycle crunches
Post-workout stretching	triceps stretches (3 minutes)
Relaxation	10 to 20 minutes

Week Three: Thursday, Friday, Saturday

Pre-workout stretching	wide-stance standing circular hip stretches (2 minutes)

Cardio exercise	squat thrusts and burpees (3 minutes each); jog in place (4 minutes)
Stretching	bent-over hamstring and lower back stretches (2 minutes each)
Strength training	Starting with the number you can comfortably complete, work up to:
	50 lunges
	70 body squats
	50 dips
	50 pull-ups
	50 calf raises (25 each leg)
Post-workout stretching	seated cross-leg toe touches (2 minutes)
Relaxation	10 to 20 minutes

Week Four: Monday, Wednesday, Friday

Pre-workout stretching	15 vertical jumps
Cardio exercise	jogging in place (5 minutes)
Stretching	50 jumping jacks
Strength training	Starting with the number you can comfortably complete, work up to:
	75 jump squats
	50 lunges
	50 dips
	50 Indian push-ups
	50 leg raises
Post-workout stretching	50 arm spins
Relaxation	10 to 20 minutes

Week Four: Tuesday, Thursday, Saturday

Pre-workout stretching	25 jumping jacks
Cardio exercise	stair jogging (5 minutes)
Stretching	50 windmills

Strength training	Starting with the number you can comfortably complete, work up to:
	60 push-ups
	60 pull-ups
	10 chin-ups
	70 calf raises (35 each leg)
Post-workout stretching	door jamb stretches (3 minutes)
Relaxation	10 to 20 minutes

Checking-In with Dave, Our Health and Fitness Entrepreneur

In Chapter Three, we mentioned that we'd check-in with Dave in this chapter, after he'd had time to practice his health and fitness routine as a frequent business traveler.

What Dave has discovered is that he sometimes has business trips that, for one reason or another, throw him off his health and fitness routine. But he knows that it's the cumulative effect of his healthy routines that counts, not a few missed exercise sessions, or a few less-than-ideal meals. And so Dave returns to his complete health and fitness routine as soon as he can, knowing how much better he feels when he does, which is also a huge incentive.

What's the big-picture pay off?

Following his health and fitness plan means that Dave is able to do his job without sacrificing his health. And it means that he can engage in frequent business travel while maintaining a level of fitness that continues to improve every six months or so. He's been pleasantly surprised by how much of a difference he can make in his own physical well-being, just by following the guidelines he worked out with his travel fitness coach and his nutritionist.

In Chapter Five, we'll check-in with Ed, too, as he completes his first year as a frequent business traveler.

Chapter 5: On and Off the Road: Your Lifetime Health and Fitness Commitment

You no doubt have a pretty good idea of where you'd like to course-correct your FBT work life—to improve, if not maximize, your overall health and fitness. So what's the best way to make a lasting commitment to your long-term well-being, both on and off the road?

Starting from Scratch

You may have decided that you need to start from scratch, like Bob, our Health and Fitness Start-up Hero. Remember how, even though Bob began his FBT job in relatively good physical shape, after six years on the road (six years of consuming airport/airline/restaurant food, and living a stressful but sedentary life), he'd gained thirty-two pounds and acquired high blood pressure, high cholesterol, and elevated blood sugar?

And how, when Bob recovered from the shock of hearing his physician's findings about his health (three incipient chronic illnesses, in addition to all that extra weight), he realized that the solution was really not so complex?

All he needed to repair the damage his job had done, was a workable on-the-road exercise plan, and strategies for obtaining nutritionally balanced, healthy meal, in places not widely noted for serving them.

To pursue both goals, Bob hired a personal health and fitness trainer, and started to improve his health with small steps. He learned how to make better food choices, while also teaching himself to incorporate exercise into odd moments throughout his day. After that, over the course of several months, Bob gradually found ways to incorporate cardio workouts, strength training, and stretching into his daily schedule.

Though none of his efforts were the slightest bit superhuman, he was astonished at how successful they were. A mere four months later, Bob's doctor was happy to report that he'd lost ten pounds, and that each of his incipient chronic conditions had disappeared. His blood pressure, cholesterol, and blood sugar had all returned to normal.

So if you, like Bob, have neglected most aspects of your health, it's certainly not impossible—and not all that difficult— to turn things around, and to do so in a relatively short time. But it's best to start with a medical exam, so you know whether or not you need to exercise with a medical condition in mind. It's also a good idea to get professional help in setting up your new health program, at least in the beginning.

Planning for Success

What if your situation is more like that of Dave, our Health and Fitness Entrepreneur?

Here is someone who exercised regularly and ate healthy meals when he was at home, but found it difficult to do either when traveling for his job. And yet, because Dave didn't like what a mere five months as an FBT had done to his health and well-being, he eventually turned to experts (a travel fitness coach and a nutritionist) to help him preplan exercise and healthy meals, and offer their ongoing support, while he reformed his daily habits on the road.

In the end, Dave scheduled his time to accommodate early morning exercises and stress-reduction routines. He also committed to filling out his health journal, a daily record of everything he ate and every exercise repetition he did. More than anything else, Dave's journal helped him see where he was making progress, and where he still needed to improve his daily routines and, ultimately, to restore his health.

If you're in a place in your FBT work life that is similar to Dave's before he sought professional assistance, then you are sufficiently fit to exercise without difficulty, and you know the difference between faux food and healthy meals.

All you actually need is a little assistance in incorporating healthier routines into your FBT work life. And even though it's true that you could probably come up with a good plan by yourself, it's still wise to hire an expert, someone knowledgeable, whom you'll have to be accountable to. That's because the temptation to start "later" or "after next month" is too great, especially when you're trying to catch flights, get to multiple meetings in a single day, and close deals in record time. Your body, however, can't wait. It needs good nutrition and regular exercise. And it needs them right now, today.

Health and Fitness as Valuable Business Assets

If neither Bob's nor Dave's challenges resemble where you are in managing your FBT work life, it could be that you are a bit more like Ed, our Health and Fitness CEO.

For Ed, physical fitness, health, and well-being are a kind of second job. That's because Ed knows all his career accomplishments are at least partially the result of his high-level physical health (which translates into mental and emotional health, as well), and which he works to build and maintain each day.

In fact, as a result of Ed's commitment to his health "vocation," he has spent time, over the years, helping his company understand the role that physical fitness plays in what they value about him most: his ability to structure and close impossible deals that no one else can. And so, when his company wanted him to take a FBT job, he lobbied for and got special benefits as part of his employment contract. Those benefits help Ed maintain his health on the road, and they include the ability to arrive two days early, stay two days late, get a room with a kitchenette, and only stay in hotels with a gym and a pool on the premises.

Ed's company might not be willing to provide all those benefits for someone they considered less critical to their business goals. But Ed had earned substantial leverage over the years, and he brought that leverage to bear in negotiating working conditions which help him maintain his health, while also doing critical work for his company. As his company immediately recognized, it's a benefit to both of them, a win-win deal.

Of course, not everyone has the leverage to get job benefits like Ed's. Still, there are ways to plan your FBT work life so you can get the exercise and healthy meals you need. And who knows? If you can make a convincing case for your health and fitness as a job asset, your company, like Ed's, may be willing to offer at least a few concessions to make your FBT work life a healthier experience.

Wherever you are, though, relative to restoring your health as a frequent business traveler, one thing is certain. Doing everything you can to build and maintain every aspect of your physical, mental, and emotional fitness—both on the road and off, as well as throughout your lifetime—is well worth it.

Why Health and Fitness Support Every Aspect of Your Life

Why are health and fitness worthwhile as present, future, and lifetime goals? There are many good reasons.

Your Longevity Is at Stake

Statistically speaking, men die five years earlier than women, having a life expectancy, at present, of seventy-five, as opposed to the statistical average for women, which is eighty. But you don't have to succumb to statistics. You can significantly improve your longevity by gradually building and maintaining your health and fitness, starting right now.

Your Job Is at Stake

As mentioned in Chapter Four, being a road warrior is akin to being an athlete. The strenuous and typically stressful nature of working on the road means that the physical demands, and the mental, emotional, and psychological flexibility required for success, are substantial. So when you make the extra effort to eat a nutritious diet and get daily exercise, you are making it possible for your body to help you do your FBT job—and continue to do it, for as long as you wish.

Eating poorly and getting little or no exercise, on the other hand, mean that you'll have a much harder time doing your job. You'll also be far more likely to develop one or more chronic illnesses, in addition to the probability that you'll gain more and more weight, the longer you travel for business. Remember that statistic mentioned at the beginning of this book, that 90 percent of all FBTs eventually become obese?

Your Quality of Life Is at Stake
Your body knows the difference between healthy food and fake food products that contain the high six: high-fat; high-sugar; high-salt; high-calories; high-carbs (simple, not complex carbohydrates); and highly processed and chemicalized. Your body also knows the difference between a well-exercised, vibrant version of itself, and a sedentary, lethargic version.

To feel truly alive—physically, emotionally, and mentally—good nutrition and the vitality that comes from daily exercise are not only essential, they're also the only way to achieve that healthy, vital state.

A Big Overall Difference Is at Stake
There are many specific benefits that come from cultivating the habit of good nutrition and daily exercise, and they range from lower cholesterol to more restful sleep. Here is a complete list:
• A general feeling of well-being
• All your systems of elimination (lungs, sweat glands, lymph glands, bloodstream, liver, digestive tract, kidneys) detoxify your body more efficiently
• An easier time quieting the "fight or flight" response of the sympathetic nervous system, while more easily wakening the parasympathetic nervous system, which is responsible for relaxing the muscles, dilating the blood vessels, and restoring the endocrine system to normal
• If you have type 2 diabetes, you may be able to gradually manage it

without medication; if you are prediabetic, you may be able to gradually overcome the insulin resistance that leads to diabetes

• A stronger immune system because of an increase in white blood cells and corticosteroid production, which enhances your ability to deal with allergies, and lessens your risk of some kinds of cancer

• If you have high blood pressure, you may be able to gradually restore it to normal

• A reduced likelihood of myocardial infarction (heart attack), because the conditions leading up to it are reduced and often eliminated with good nutrition and daily exercise

• A reduced presence of "bad" cholesterol, or LDL, that can clog your arteries and lead to a heart attack

• Aerobic capacity, or an increased tolerance for vigorous exercise, is greatly enhanced, at the same time that your respiratory tract gets cleared and cleansed

• A reduction in headaches due to muscle tension or digestive upset, with a corresponding enhancement of the functioning of your lower digestive tract or bowel

• A reduction in excess body fat

• The diminished dysfunction or actual healing of your musculoskeletal system, as your joints and bones come into proper alignment, due to regular exercise

• Aerobic activity sends more oxygen to your brain, which means your mind will be clearer and work more efficiently

• Good nutrition and daily exercise yield more overall energy (in addition to a reduction in depression, negative thinking, and lethargy), and an enhanced libido resulting from good health and vital energy

• Vigorous exercise leads to a release of endorphins, the brain's natural opiate, which produces a gentle high, or feeling of well-being that can last up to an hour or more

• The ability to get to sleep quickly, and to experience deep, restful sleep, nightly

Can You Recognize Good Health and Fitness When You See It?

It's not as simple as it seems. Overall health, fitness, and mental well-being involve seven key elements that require both daily attention and long-term cultivation or nurturance:

1. Cardiovascular conditioning from aerobic exercise

2. Muscular development from strength training using resistance such as exercise or weights

3. Musculoskeletal flexibility, or stretching and lengthening the muscles, ligaments, and tendons for greater flexibility and overall healthfulness

4. Core strength from strengthening the abdominal muscles, pelvic floor muscles, and the muscles of the back on either side of the spine

5. Healthy nutrition from a diet of vegetables, fruits, grains, beans, nuts and seeds, and optional light animal protein (fish, eggs, chicken) in moderation, along with vitamin supplements

6. Periods of mental relaxation from regular time spent practicing the relaxation response and/or meditating

7. Nightly sleep—between seven and nine hours

If you focus your efforts on enhancing each of these health components, daily, you will achieve better cardiovascular conditioning, greater large-muscle strength, more musculoskeletal flexibility, increased core muscle strength, improved nutritional health, greater mental calm, improved overall restfulness, and greater sleep sufficiency, gradually and over time. You'll also cover all the bases for achieving health and fitness.

Let's take a closer look at each of the seven areas that together comprise your optimal level of both health and fitness.

Cardiovascular Conditioning

Aerobic exercise (that is, exercise designed to increase your intake of oxygen, because it's strenuous enough to produce deeper, faster breathing) is an excellent way to give your heart muscle and circulatory system the workout it needs to become healthier, while also achieving a state of optimal conditioning.

To succeed at cardiovascular conditioning, the exercise you do should increase your heart rate. The goal is to raise your heartbeat so that your beats-per-minute represent 50 to 70 percent of your heart's maximum rate (calculated according to your age), for a moderate intensity workout. For a vigorous intensity workout, the rate should be 70 to 85 percent,.

You can figure your maximum heart rate by subtracting your age from two hundred and twenty (for example, 220 minus 38 years of age would be 182 beats per minute). To figure the percentages for a moderate workout or a vigorous one, multiply your maximum heart rate by 0.50 and 0.70, for a moderate workout, or by 0.70 and 0.85, for a vigorous one (182 x 0.50 = 91; 182 x 0.70 = 127.40; 182 x 0.85 = 154.7). The resulting number is the number of heartbeats per minute that you need to attain and maintain to get the workout you want. This is also known as your target heart rate. You should keep your heart pumping at your target rate for a minimum of twenty minutes to have the desired workout effect. You should build up to that time period, of course, depending on your starting level of fitness.

But whether your workout is moderate or vigorous, it will have the same result: Over time, you'll achieve higher levels of cardiovascular conditioning. The benefits of such conditioning are similar to most health and fitness regimes; that is, a loss of excess weight; a stronger heart muscle; lower blood pressure; reduced "bad" or LDL cholesterol; a diminished risk of heart attack; and normalized blood sugar.

Muscular Development

Strength training, or increasing the size of all the large muscle groups by either lifting weights or pulling against (resisting) weight, is important to overall fitness, for a number of reasons.

First, after the age of twenty, men lose half a pound of muscle mass every year, if muscle building isn't part of their daily and weekly routine. That rate of lost muscle mass actually doubles after the age of sixty.

But there are other good reasons to build muscle strength. Stronger, larger muscles increase your metabolism (the rate at which you burn calories), and make it easier to lose weight. Strengthening the large muscles also increases bone density, which reduces the risk of fractures due to bone weakness. Muscle fitness improves the function of your heart, too, while elevating your "good" (HDL) cholesterol.

In other words, building strong muscles does a lot more for you than what you see in the mirror.

Musculoskeletal Flexibility

Physical flexibility comes from adding a comprehensive stretching routine to your daily workout. Lengthening your muscles, ligaments, and tendons by extending your limbs and bending in all directions, while holding those positions for up to a minute, helps you elongate and stretch them. This is the opposite of what weight training and aerobic exercise do; that is, they contract and shorten them. And when your muscles are "tight" because of contraction, your posture suffers and you risk injury due to a lack of musculoskeletal flexibility. Stretching not only counteracts that tendency, it restores and improves your range of motion. In turn, that flexibility allows your legs and arms to move within their joints more easily, and prevents falls or other accidents because you enjoy much better balance with a normalized range of motion.

But that's not all. Stretching also alleviates mental stress stored in your body as muscle tension, improves your circulation, and sends fresh oxygen to muscles that are oxygen deprived.

What is more heartening, perhaps, is that you only need to hold a stretch for thirty to sixty seconds to get the benefits you're looking for. Don't "bounce" in a stretch position; just stretch and hold, for up to a minute. Also, don't overstretch, or stretch to the point of pain. This isn't beneficial, and could even result in an injury. Stretching should be a pain-free exercise, one in which there is no pain but a definite net gain.

Core Strength

Strengthening all the muscles that comprise your core—your abdominal muscles, the muscles of your pelvic floor, and the muscles of your back on either side of your spine—is important for a whole host of reasons.

These core muscles are the reason you are able to complete everyday tasks with ease and assurance. Task like bending, turning around, sitting up straight in a chair, getting dressed, taking a shower, standing tall, and maintaining good posture all depend on your core muscles.. They're also why you can enjoy sports and even sexual activity. Golf, tennis, biking, running, swimming, and so forth, all rely on your core muscles, as does sexual activity.

Healthy Nutrition

As we saw in Chapter Two, in particular, your health and fitness depend upon the quality of the food you habitually consume. You've probably heard that old saying about the way computers operate: "Garbage in. Garbage out." A computer can only produce results relative to the quality of the data it has been "fed." And the same concept applies to your nutrition. If you eat highly processed food that is laden with high-fructose corn syrup, trans fat, salt, and chemicals of all kinds, you are going to produce a body that is running on empty calories and isn't getting the nutrients it needs—a body that is, in effect, starving. No wonder it breaks down. Sooner, if not later.

Working in the extremely strenuous world of frequent business travel, you need even better nutrition, not the absolute worst food typically available in airports, on airplanes, and in many restaurants.

These days, it is widely accepted that a diet built around food that's as close as possible to its natural state (unprocessed food, in other words) is far better for your health than ultra-preserved, ultra-processed faux food that is dead in terms of its nutritional value. To get the best physical results, then, create an on-the-road diet that offers lots of vegetables and fruits (preferably organic, or pesticide-free); grains; beans;

nuts and seeds; and finally, organically produced light animal protein, like eggs, fish, and chicken. Stay away from red meat, processed meats, and meat in general, as these are known to produce artery-clogging plaque.

The myth that athletes, in particular, and people, in general, need to get protein from red meat is starting to fade in the public awareness, and even in the not-especially-healthy mainstream media, too. That is the result of many things, but could also be due to the fact that more athletes of all types are turning to vegetarian and even vegan diets. These diets give athletes the complex nutrients they need for high-level physical functioning without all the unhealthy stuff associated with traditional meat-potatoes-and-dessert diets (for more on this topic, simply Google "vegetarian and vegan athletes").

What these athletes (from professional football players to world class ironman triathletes) have discovered confirms the nutritional recommendations made by Harvard researchers. In Chapter Two, you may remember, we explored the research conducted by the Harvard School of Public Health in some detail. But in its simplest form, the Harvard nutritional guidelines call for meals centered around vegetables (as the largest portion); followed by whole grains; healthy oils (vegetable oils like olive, canola, soy, sunflower); healthy protein (fish, poultry, eggs, beans, tofu, nuts, seeds); and fruits, plus water (milk or other dairy products are not recommended for daily consumption). And for most people, a non-synthetic multivitamin and extra vitamin D are also recommended.

The Harvard guidelines are based on scientific evidence, not, as with the guidelines recommended by the USDA, on political pressure from various food industry lobbies. They offer frequent business travelers healthy meals with all the complex nutrients, carbohydrates, and protein they need to do a strenuous, often-stressful job with relative ease.

Periods of Mental Relaxation

Just as your body can become so tired it doesn't function well after hours spent flying between continents, followed by non-stop meetings, your mind, too, can become so tired and overworked that it becomes inefficient. When that happens—or better yet, before it does— it's wise to spend an hour or so "unplugging" from work and stress, and relaxing your mind. Think you're too busy to do that? Here are some good reasons to reconsider:

• Mental and physical stress can leave your immune system compromised, making you more vulnerable to illness, like the common cold, or worse, because airplanes are breeding grounds for contagion.

• Mental overload is not healthy for your heart, and putting extra stress on that essential muscle can compromise all your bodily systems.

• Stress and overload both tend to compromise the ability to remember things (not useful for important meetings), and they also make it more difficult to make good decisions.

• Mental overload and stress increase the risk of a stroke.

• Ironically, mental overload and its accompanying stress make you more vulnerable to depression and negative thinking.

• When in a stressed or mentally overloaded state, your stress hormone, cortisol, is released in larger amounts. Because cortisol stimulates your appetite—particularly the craving for salty, fatty, or sweet junk food— it can actually cause weight gain

So there are many good reasons to give your mind a rest and prevent mental stress burnout.

A detailed discussion of the relaxation response—what it is, how to induce it—appears in Chapter Three. Rather than repeat that information here, suffice it to say that the benefits of mental relaxation are similar, although a bit less dramatic, to those resulting from actual meditation (a topic also discussed in that chapter). But the benefits, as you might expect, are largely the flip side of the above detrimental effects caused by mental stress, and they include:

• Restoring your immune system's ability to fight off illness or infection

- De-stressing your heart
- Restoring your normal memory and decision-making ability
- Diminished risk of stroke
- Decreased vulnerability to depression and negative thinking
- Decrease in the amount of cortisol, the stress hormone, circulating in your system, and a corresponding normalization of your appetite

For its part, meditation adds a deeper dimension to the above positive effects. It results in not just an enhancement of memory and the ability to focus, but an increase in creativity and feelings of compassion. To achieve the latter two results, a meditator need only devote about twenty minutes each day—focusing solely on one thought, word, or image —for a period as short as two to four weeks. Of course, the true benefits, including positive changes in the actual structure of the brain, can only be realized after several years of regular meditation practice.

Nightly Sleep

Sleep may be the best form of physical and mental rest and healing that's available to you, under normal circumstances. It certainly ranks with air, food, and water as an essential for sustaining human life. All the detrimental effects that result from poor nutrition, stress, and lack of exercise also show up when you suffer from a lack of sleep. In other words, if you don't get enough sleep, you open yourself up to immune dysfunction, heart stress, stroke risk, stress that's unalleviated, loss of memory, loss of the ability to focus and pay attention, weight gain, risk of diabetes, and mood disorders.

Adults need between seven and nine hours of sleep each night to repair and rebuild their bodies, improve their immune function, and organize and process information accumulated during the waking state. The Harvard Medical School's Division of Sleep Medicine has conducted research showing how vital a role sleep plays in maintaining physical health, emotional well-being, and even in fostering longevity.

Everyone feels better after a good night's sleep, but that's not all that sleep offers. Solutions to problems that stumped you yesterday may suddenly reveal themselves the next morning, as your mind was busy working on them while you slept. Physical and mental rest and repair—and solutions, too. Who could ask for anything more?

Health and Fitness Common Sense

The bottom line on health and fitness is simply a matter of common sense.

When you work toward ever-higher levels of both, you are giving your body the nutrition, exercise, relaxation time, and sleep it needs to function optimally.

And not just on the road, or for the time you spend doing your job, but throughout your entire lifetime.

As we've just seen, it is well worth it.

* 9 7 8 0 9 9 0 3 0 9 4 4 4 *